THE VITAMIN CURE

for Depression

BO H. JONSSON, M.D., PH.D.
AND ANDREW W. SAUL, PH.D.

Basic Health
PUBLICATIONS, INC.

The information contained in this book is based upon the research and personal and professional experiences of the authors. It is not intended as a substitute for consulting with your physician or other healthcare provider. Any attempt to diagnose and treat an illness should be done under the direction of a healthcare professional.

The publisher does not advocate the use of any particular healthcare protocol but believes the information in this book should be available to the public. The publisher and authors are not responsible for any adverse effects or consequences resulting from the use of the suggestions, preparations, or procedures discussed in this book. Should the reader have any questions concerning the appropriateness of any procedures or preparation mentioned, the authors and the publisher strongly suggest consulting a professional healthcare advisor.

Basic Health Publications, Inc.

www.basichealthpub.com

Library of Congress Cataloging-in-Publication Data is available through the Library of Congress.

Jonsson, Bo H.
    The vitamin cure for depression : orthomolecular treatment of depression / Bo H. Jonsson, M.D., Ph.D., and Andrew W. Saul, Ph.D.
        pages cm
    Includes bibliographical references and index.
    ISBN 978-1-59120-282-0 (alk. paper)
    1. Depression, Mental—Chemotherapy. 2. Vitamin therapy. I. Saul, Andrew W. II. Title.
    RC537.J67   2012
    616.85'27061—dc23

                                                    2012038641

Editor: Karen Anspach
Typesetting/Book design: Gary A. Rosenberg
Cover design: Mike Stromberg

Printed in the United States of America

10   9   8   7   6   5   4   3   2   1

CONTENTS

CONTENTS

ACKNOWLEDGEMENTS

During the last ten years some doctors were especially important for me to find and join in the orthomolecular movement. They were first David Horrobin and the Swedish psychiatrist Per Dalén. Later on, I was inspired by Karin Munsterhjelm and Harold Foster. In 2004 I read a scientific paper, just published, written by Abram Hoffer. My first reaction was that it could not be the same Abram Hoffer who, more than fifty years earlier, found that some patients with schizophrenia were cured with niacin and in the 1960s had inspired Linus Pauling, who coined the word orthomolecular. But it was, and the following year we met in person. My parents, many teachers, colleagues, friends, my two daughters, and my darling companion Regina have all been most important for my sail.

—BO H. JONSSON

As colleagues and as friends, orthomolecular psychiatrists Abram Hoffer and Hugh D. Riordan taught me how well nutritional medicine really works. I thank my own personal support team, consisting primarily of my daughter Helen, my son Jason, my longtime undergrad-to-doctoral mentor Dr. John I. Mosher, and the two most expert counselors I ever met: James Hughes and Richard Bennett. I also thank my much better half, Colleen, for having a *real* job and thus making this book possible. May I add that I think I have found an excellent depression preventive: my granddaughter.

—ANDREW W. SAUL

Both authors would like to thank the International Schizophrenia Foundation, the *Journal of Orthomolecular Medicine,* and all the writers and peer-reviewers of the *Orthomolecular Medicine News Service.* Our thanks also go to Dr. Jonathan Prousky, Steven Carter, Mike Stewart, and Robert Sarver. We especially thank Drs. Steve Hickey and Hilary Roberts for their kind permission to include their commentary on evidence-based medicine and MEDLINE, and Dr. John I. Mosher for his insightful text on lifestyle modification and stress reduction techniques.

FOREWORD

At the beginning of my work as an orthomolecular physician about twenty years ago, I had a revolutionary "aha!" experience. The ability to question the relevance of certain aspects of the medical establishment is necessary, and even essential, for doctors who work in a well-structured medical system. I had already worked for fifteen years in different hospitals and healthcare centers, and had accomplished my specialist competence in general medicine. In the Nordic countries general medicine is valid as a separate specialist competence that demands an additional examination. I thought this competence would best cover my need for a holistic view of human health.

A middle-aged woman, a cleaner, had been my patient for a long time. She visited a psychiatrist, too. She had gotten the diagnosis of fibromyalgia with medium-severe depression, and had already been on sickness benefits for many long episodes because of her great difficulties with heavy manual labor. Now the patient, the psychiatrist, and I thought it would be wise to also try to obtain a sickness pension for her. No medical proceedings had given any reasonable help—the patient was completely "worn out," as she herself pointed out. She had severe body pain, growing exhaustion ("like lead in my whole body"), a very disturbed sleep pattern, and her depression increased alarmingly. During one of our regular meetings with the patient, as we started to gather comprehensive information about her illness to complete a reliable application for the sickness pension (no easy task with these diagnoses), I had the idea that she could still try a little tablet of 100 mcg organic selenium, combined with 15 milligrams of zinc and a little dose of vitamin E, until we met again. We thought that the documents would be ready by then. I did not know much about selenium, but I knew some of its working mechanisms, including that it binds to mercury and is a strong antioxidant. I knew that our soil in the Northern European countries lacks selenium. Some weeks later the patient returned. She was very happy and told me that the little selenium pill had an unbelievable influence on her whole situation. She felt like a new human being and she wanted to return to her work! She continued to take this selenium pill (not a high dose from an orthomolecular point of view) every day and her improved health situation continued during the years I still saw her. For me, as a conventional doctor, this was really like witnessing a miracle. I had taken my first stumbling steps into a medical world that now, twenty years later, after intense researching and comprehensive clinical experience, seems to have no limits at all. This world represents a completely different view on human health and the risks of chronic illnesses compared to what I had learned earlier during all my years as a medical student and later in clinical practice.

It is surely not always that easy as with this patient. That was a real stroke of luck! During the last twenty years I have walked ever deeper into the ecological and evolutionary way of understanding human health and health-disturbances. I have also learned that this medicine is based on a strong scientific foundation that goes far back in time. It is called orthomolecular medicine, a concept that was introduced and defined by the two-time Nobel laureate Linus Pauling in his 1968 article, "Orthomolecular Psychiatry," in *Science*.

You will read much more about this in the important and comprehensive book you now have in your hands. This book is of great significance for those who suffer depression with treatment complications and who wish to seek help outside the usual medicine of today.

This book covers a surprisingly large number of different perspectives. It is a fantastic mix of genuine knowledge, interesting scientific reasoning, life wisdom, and—not to forget—humor! It presents an analysis of a selected group of the orthomolecular substances that have such a marvelous healing power, each one respectively or often even better in combinations.

You will also find many other views of primary interest for understanding human health in modern society. For example, today's food, which is sometimes nearly toxic, needs to be replaced by foods better suited to our "old" genes. This problem is thoroughly discussed and made understandable by applying evolution-based reasoning. Even if the chapters about research, science, and "evidence-based medicine" (EBM) may appear a little difficult I really want to encourage the reader to have patience and carefully go through them. They will provide interesting insight into our modern medicine and why it is so difficult to incorporate fundamental orthomolecular knowledge into our established medical system. Every physician who has worked with orthomolecular medicine for a long time and knows the convincing history of this medical approach and the scientific and clinical work of the great pioneers has asked this question many times: *How is it possible to neglect this basic medical knowledge?* How is it possible that orthomolecular medicine, which enables so many patients to recover and is so logical and easy to understand is, decade after decade, met with such resistance by the medical establishment? Why do so many colleagues look down or start talking about something else when the word vitamin is mentioned? At the same time that patient demand for these therapies just grows and grows, and the few physicians working in this medical specialty are overwhelmed with work and cries for help. Lack of knowledge can not be the only explanation! Patients and their relatives are, more and more, looking for knowledge and help on the Internet. This book gives fundamental information and explanations to what is happening.

I also like what is written about the healing power of nature. I believe that humans' alienation from a life in harmony with nature is one of the big problems of today. To be close to nature is nearly always a comfort to a sad mood. This probably is due to a combination of many factors: the eye is enjoying the beauty; the ear the silence, the song of the birds, or the wind whistling in the crowns of the trees; the sense of smell the pines and moss and clean air rich in oxygen; the sense of taste the fresh-gathered blueberries or murmuring spring water; and the sense of touch the wonderful feeling of walking barefoot through the grass or over sun-warmed rocks, or slowly swimming through soft water. Perhaps, also in such moments, our "sixth sense" is best able to open up and feel how everything is connected. Anyhow—nature gives solace in many ways, from biological, psychological, philosophical, and spiritual points of view.

As to my own career, I gradually learned more about orthomolecular medicine. I started to combine my long experience in established medicine with this new knowledge full time. I started my own practice and worked part-time at the Antioxidant Clinics that surgeon Kaarlo Jaakkola, the foremost pioneer in Finland in nutritional medicine, had started in the beginning of the 1980s. There I had contact with likeminded colleagues and access to a well-developed mineral laboratory with the ability to measure the vitamin, mineral, and fatty acid concentrations in serum and whole blood. I met well-informed patients on a daily basis who wanted to try something more than established medicine could offer. And hence my patients became my best teachers and coworkers.

A young man asked for my help. He had felt increasingly unwell for many years. He thought his diet was healthy and he tried to exercise regularly. He neither smoked nor used large quantities of alcohol. But he felt exhausted and ever more depressed, and could be overwhelmed by such states of severe weakness a couple of hours after a meal that he had to lay down, wherever he was. He had looked for help in general health care. Nothing was wrong with him and antidepressants only gave him side effects. I put him on a five-hour glucose load, but it had to be stopped after three hours because his blood sugar dropped so low that he needed something to eat immediately. He had the same feeling of weakness that he would have some hours after a meal. There was diabetes in his family. And he had experienced another situation where he felt the same way—it was at the dentist. The dentist had drilled in one of his old amalgam fillings. After that he felt very bad for many days, with headaches, nausea, vertigo, and weakness. I started by recommending a diet free from all sugars and fast carbohydrates like potato, white flour, pasta, and white rice, and increasing his intake of proteins and natural fat. He rapidly got a little bit better. Then I prescribed a combination of vitamins, minerals, and fatty acids in orthomolecular doses. He again felt better. He really started to recover when a dentist professionally skilled in amalgam replacement therapy replaced all his amalgam fillings with nontoxic material. In the patient's own opinion this was the most important step to recovery. It has been many years since then. I recently talked with the patient and he happily told me he was feeling well and was still progressing in his improvement. He continues with his nutrients and his diet. Amalgam fillings contain about 50 percent mercury, a heavy metal that is biologically very toxic. The fillings continually emit mercury vapor, a process that can be accelerated by many factors. The mercury vapor is then absorbed into the body and the brain by many means, including through the lungs and directly to the brain via the olfactory nerve. There are some individuals who have a higher sensitivity to mercury than others, and this was probably the case with my patient. Today many Scandinavian countries have forbidden the use of dental amalgam. At some point it will probably be forbidden in the whole of the European Union.

Every human being has his or her own unique biochemical profile. People don't only look different from other human beings, their inner chemical geography can also vary substantially. Maybe due to a unique set of genes a particular individual will require more of one or several nutrients than most other people, and maybe he or she will actually get sick due to this deficiency. The biochemist Roger J. Williams, Ph.D. introduced the concept *biochemical individuality,* which you can read more about in this book. This specific individuality is not only related to nutrients but also, for instance, to hormones. This means that the statistically-based normative reference ranges for hormonal blood tests are not quite valid for all patients. Some of them are sick although their laboratory values are within the standard range.

Hypothyroidism shows a multiple set of symptoms. In this group of symptoms there normally is some form of depression. This depression can be mild but it can also show up in a more extreme form, like psychosis. Today the traditional treatment medication is levothyroxine, for instance Synthroid, while another old medication, which was successfully prescribed in the past, is forgotten. Natural desiccated thyroid, for instance Armour Thyroid, was used from the beginning of the twentieth century up to some decades ago. One example of the efficiency of this natural, orthomolecular medication is the following "sunshine story."

A deeply concerned mother came to my office with her fourteen-year-old daughter. This girl had been diagnosed as hypothyroid a year ago, and was on levothyroxine treatment. All her hormone blood tests were within the "excellent" range, but the girl was evidently quite sick—I could see it when she walked through my door. Her whole appearance signaled that something was wrong. Her clothes were black, and she was fully decorated with chains and steel pins. Her hair was green and her face expressed a sullen anger. I could not talk to her; she was silent and looked down on the floor, but she allowed me to give her a physical examination. I found cold, dry skin with obvious myxedema (typical for an under-functioning thyroid) on her face and the outer side of her upper arms. Her hair was dry and straggling, and the outer third of her eyebrows were missing. Her blood pressure was low and her pulse rather accelerated. Her body temperature was low. Her mother mentioned that her daughter did not attend school anymore. At home she had severe outbreaks of rage and in between she was in bed sleeping or crying. She was obviously hypothyroid in spite of the good labs. She was in a bad state and actually needed hospital care, but her mother was very much determined. She wanted her daughter to try Armour Thyroid, which she had read about. Since her mother had the option to stay at home and look after her daughter I agreed to try this, along with frequent visits to me as a control. There are not many doctors today who know this old medication of desiccated thyroid, but I have found that this natural medication often works much better than levothyroxine for my patients. The girl quickly improved and already after a month she was back in school. After a year she was like any normal teenager. She managed very well at school and talked to me with an open mind and clear insight. She dressed like most teenagers. The recovery has been stable.

I am convinced that many suicides could be avoided and deep depressions could heal more quickly and more thoroughly or be prevented if treated correctly. This could be the case given one important condition: that the very broad view of these illnesses, their etiology, prevention, and treatment, as presented in this book, is taken into account.

I will end my foreword with the last lines in the magnificent little book, *Darkness Visible: A Memoir of Madness,* written by the many time award-winning American author William Styron. It has nothing to do with orthomolecular medicine but describes in a deeply reflective and naked way the author's own path through a deep depression, where the danger of suicide was immediate. He refers at the end of his book to Dante's *Divina Commedia* and ends with the beautiful words:

> For those who have dwelt in depression's dark wood, and know its inexplicable agony, their return from the abyss is not unlike the ascent of the poet, trudging upward and upward out of hell's black depths and at last emerging into what he saw as "the shining world." There, whoever has been restored to health has almost always been restored to the capacity for serenity and joy, and this may be indemnity enough for having endured the despair beyond despair.
>
> *E quindi uscimmo a riveder le stelle.*
> And so we came forth, and once again beheld the stars.

—KARIN MUNSTERHJELM-AHUMADA, M.D.

PREFACE

HOW I GOT INTO NUTRITIONAL MEDICINE

The first time I (BHJ) came across the statement that vitamins could be effective as treatment for psychiatric disease was during the early 1970s, when I was in medical school. It was not discussed in any lecture and no one ever mentioned it. The information I found was in books and journals I sought out myself. For some reason I had an interest in natural treatments, possibly directed at the origin of disease.

That psychiatric disease can be comprehended in evolutionary terms or that it can be highly dependent on lifestyle factors was seldom taught. The understanding of psychiatric disease was mainly based on symptoms and behavior. The origin of disease was little known and was abstractly described as related to genetics and some environmental aspects. Psychosocial factors and trauma were often emphasized, while other environmental factors such as food and environmental toxins were unspecified or neglected. If considered at all, any description of underlying pathophysiology or biochemistry was often superficial and biased, with a pharmacological drug perspective. The prognosis of psychiatric disease was usually pessimistic. The best option was considered to be treatment with drugs, but the truth was that for many people with depression current medical treatments were (and are) less than optimal. During the 1980s I specialized in general psychiatry, working as a doctor in the emergency room, in hospital inpatient wards, and in outpatient facilities. I met all kinds of patients, their diagnoses labeled schizophrenia, manic or bipolar depression, unipolar depression, and anxiety syndromes, as well as borderline and other personality disturbances or complicated stress disorders. Many of them had alcohol or other substance abuse. Main treatment alternatives were pharmacological drugs, psychotherapy, and limited social intervention measures.

Having worked some years as a psychiatrist I noticed that the results in clinical work were often less successful than those described in books and scientific papers highly influenced by pharmaceutical industry. Some of my colleagues made similar observations. Commonly, patients receiving antidepressant drugs suffered from side effects, and many received no certain or insufficient results. Also, a lot of patients got better without drugs or specific psychotherapy. After many years I realized that often the most effective treatment and best results were obtained not by following what the textbooks, teachers, experts, or authorities told me, but rather by finding out for myself, making decisions, and cooperating with each patient individually.

During the 1990s I worked in stress research at the Karolinska Institutet, which resulted in a dissertation in 1999. My view of modern medicine evolved into a more critical perspective. It became clear that part of what generally was called science was little more than opinion, sometimes prejudiced. What was labeled evidence-based medicine was still mostly authoritarian-based medicine. A good working alliance involving the patient is important. Applying direct observation and critical thinking during the patient visit is a small scientific task. Conventional psychiatric medical knowledge today needs integration with an understanding of the role of food and nutrition, sleep, light and physical outdoor activity, cultural and environmental factors, stress management, and a positive attitude. Each patient needs individual evaluation and treatment determined specifically for them. I found that several of my patients clearly benefitted from this holistic approach compared with their previous treatments.

Ten years ago a father phoned me explaining that his son had been diagnosed with schizophrenia. He wanted to know if I could help with orthomolecular treatment. I answered that unfortunately I knew very little about orthomolecular medicine, which uses a holistic approach to healing that focuses on optimal nutritional intake including supplements. A couple of years later (and thirty years after my first reading about the original research by Abram Hoffer and Humphry Osmond) I brushed up my knowledge on the specific biochemical mechanisms that may explain why optimal doses with vitamins and other nutrients can have a decisive effect in disease treatment and prevention. I found that contrary to the general belief of traditional medical professionals, the original scientific literature in the field was quite often of good or at least acceptable quality, while some of the later antivitamin literature was surprisingly devoid of scientific observation or critical and logical thinking. I started to test nutritional approaches with some of my patients, finding it sometimes made a difference.

Summing up my three decades of clinical work as a doctor I would say that during the first decade I learned to be a doctor. During the second decade I added critical thinking from my research experience. And during the last ten years I practiced and integrated knowledge from orthomolecular medicine.

I want to emphasize that conventional psychiatry with drugs and psychotherapy help lots of people. However, treatment and prevention of disease is best if all available knowledge is integrated and applied with sound judgment.

In serious, deep, long-standing, or recurrent depressions patients can benefit from contact with a doctor. But even if it is a fine contact, the patient will have to make important decisions. For this, knowledge is needed. This book is about the options for vitamins, other nutrients, and further lifestyle factors that can be implemented in an integrated treatment of depression. The field of orthomolecular medicine is vast. This book is at best a small contribution to it. It is not a systematic review—rather, its purpose is to explain how the fields of depression and orthomolecular medicine can be brought together to help patients. My hope is to inspire further inquiry, testing, and practice. Specific personal suggestions for treatment and prevention cannot be given here. Since we are all biochemically different, personal evaluation is always needed for a specific patient.

Lifestyle is important. What we eat and drink, what we think and do, are essential for recovery. In the acute state it may be that the ability to help oneself is limited. In the long run there are many paths to discover, study, and test. Working with a doctor, therapist, or other professional in a good alliance is important. Depression is not necessarily a chronic illness, but it is a tough challenge. However, finding the origins and mechanisms of depression is a most rewarding task, both for patients and professionals.

Depression and bipolar disorder are grouped together in what are called the affective disorders. This book is primarily about depression (sometimes called unipolar depression). However, because of the increase in diagnosis and labeling of bipolar disorder (manic-depressive illness), it will also be discussed in a separate chapter.

—BO H JONSSON

HOW IT ALL BEGAN FOR ME

"This boy is Ignorance. This girl is Want.
Beware them both, but most of all beware this boy."
—CHARLES DICKENS, *A CHRISTMAS CAROL*

You have just heard from an experienced, and in my opinion, brilliant orthomolecular psychiatrist. My (AWS) opinion of my coauthor was shared by our mutual late mentor, Abram Hoffer, M.D., who invariably spoke of Dr. Jonsson in the highest possible terms. I am fortunate to have benefited from my association with both of these excellent doctors. I am not a psychiatrist, I am not a physician, and I am not a research scientist. My background is in education and counseling. And, although I have over thirty years' experience in writing, lecturing, and consulting, you may consider me a wounded healer. Yes, I have worked with a considerable number of depressed people. I also have personally been through the depths of depression.

I recall (and am unlikely to forget) the very day and hour that I bottomed out. One hesitates to say that things cannot get worse, because perhaps they always can. But on that particular day in 1996, I simply could not go any lower. What did I do? I did what is now contained in this book you are reading. It worked for me. It was not instant success, it was not absolute success, and it certainly was not effortless success. It simply worked, and the more I did it the better things got. There is no monotherapy, no single magic bullet, for depression. It would be nice to make this book into a little pamphlet directing you to a single pill that you could take, get quickly cured, and be done with it. Such a tablet does not exist. There is no one drug, or cocktail of drugs, that will do the trick. Dr. Hoffer said, "Drugs make a well person sick. Why would they make a sick person well?" He added, based on his fifty-five years of psychiatric research and practice, that drug-only cure rates are about 10 percent. Optimum nutritional therapy (orthomolecular medicine) and related measures, Dr. Hoffer said, will get you an 80 percent cure rate. I like those odds.

One of the problems with depression drug therapy is that it is successful . . . for a while. Many a Prozac'ed patient will report swift and genuine improvement. Yet *maintained* selective serotonin reuptake inhibitor (SSRI) drug use can be reliably expected to cause problems down the road. This applies to antidepressant drugs in general. The bloom is off the rose all too often, as the patient reports decreasing benefit and increasing side effects. This book offers a serious alternative.

You are going to hear more of my personal story later in Chapter 11. First, we are going to present what we think will help you to better understand what depression is, why you feel the way you do, and especially what you can do about it using nutritional methods. As actress Margot Kidder said so well, "You can fix your brain with nutrition."

—ANDREW W. SAUL

INTRODUCTION

If you suffer from depression, the first good news is that this book is short. If you suffer from severe depression, this book may appear a bit too short. This is not an encyclopedia of depression. It is not even close. No book, not even a thick, comprehensive book, is enough. We do not want you to work on this alone. One of the authors is a psychiatrist; the other, an educator. You will not be surprised that we recommend that you work with a counselor and also with your physician.

Now for more good news: What we focus on in this book are nutritional treatments for depression. They are remarkably simple, safe, and easy to try. This does not mean that nutrition and depression and medicine are simple subjects. You do not need to know it all to get good results. Automobiles are very complex, yet you do not even need a high school diploma to operate one safely and efficiently. The human body is unbelievably complex, yet there are certain key areas of opportunity that are straightforward and doable. The odd thing is that so many people suffering from depression have never been encouraged, or even informed, about nutritional (orthomolecular) medicine. We'd like to fix that right now.

There are fifty-two cards in a deck. You do not need to have all of them to win at poker. Four aces will do it just fine. Four cards constitute only 8 percent of available cards. The trick is how to come up with those four. I (AWS) had a rather brief career as a professional magician. At age twelve, I was paid five dollars to perform at a birthday party. For a kid in my neighborhood in 1967, that was a lot of money.

In case you think that was an easy gig, you are mistaken. Kids are the hardest audience of all.

There is no way I would ever go to a casino unless they let me use my own cards. They will not, of course. Still, I would never place a bet unless I could stack the deck. To do so, you do not need to know how to manufacture playing cards, or the mathematical theorems of probability, or even be honest. However, you do need good technique. To beat depression, you need to stack the deck. Nutritional therapy is a really good technique. We want to show you how to use it.

ONE READER WRITES:

I just wanted to send you a sincere thank you for the information you have given me to fight my depression and anxiety the natural way. I'm twenty years old now, but my depression started when I was in seventh grade. I went to the doctor at age eighteen and I was diagnosed with bipolar, depression, and anxiety. I was on Lamictal and Wellbutrin for two years, and I just wasn't seeing any improvement. I weaned myself off the medicine and found myself feeling even worse for the next year. Two weeks ago I changed my life. In the past two weeks I've changed my diet to mostly raw foods, and started taking a multivitamin, B_{12}, and 300 milligrams of niacin a day. I feel like the person I've always wanted to be. I went out last week for the first time in a year. I've literally been too scared to leave the house, being bombarded with terrible social anxiety. It's all gone away. I feel more productive and energized then I ever have in my life. I just wish I would have found out sooner, and not had to suffer for the last eight years. Thank you for changing my outlook on life.

PART ONE

UNDERSTANDING

CHAPTER 1

THE PLAGUE OF DEPRESSION

"Doubt everything or believe everything:
these are two equally convenient strategies.
With either we dispense with the need for reflection."
—HENRI POINCARÉ (1854–1912)

During the last century depression has become more common. Is it because the disease really got more prevalent? Do depressed people seek health care more often? Do doctors diagnose depression more often? Could it be an effect of more, and perhaps better, medical treatments? Has it increased because of direct-to-consumer (DTC) drug advertisements in popular media or other forms of propaganda? These are all valid possibilities.

NATURAL REACTION AND CIVILIZATION DISEASE

Depression may be interpreted as a pure psychiatric disease, or related to a somatic disease, or a reaction to an external event. Sometimes we find no explanation. In spite of this, it is natural to talk about disease when symptoms and functional problems are severe enough. The prevalence and costs of depression are increasing globally. According to a World Health Organization study, depression was the fourth leading cause of global ill-health in 1990. It predicted that depression would be in second place, after ischemic heart disease, by 2020.[1] Even if some studies showed no difference over time, depressive disease increased overall during the twentieth century.[2] It may be that this increase is greatest for light and medium depressions, while deeper depressions are perhaps less common.[3] International research describes depression in young people as more common after World War II.[4]

Depression in Historic Times

People with depressive states have been described since ancient times. How common or rare depressions were long time ago is not known. Systematic studies of depressions in indigenous people have not been carried out. However, some authors have stated that depressions were less common among hunter-gatherers.[5] In this connection it is of interest that at least some diseases that currently can coexist with depression were less common or even unknown in earlier societies: cardiovascular disease, type 2 diabetes, and osteoporosis. Also, it can be difficult to form an understanding for the concept of "depression" as it existed in the past, as the meaning of the word has changed over time.

Categorizing the Symptoms and Origin of Depression

Current psychiatric diagnostic systems, known as The Diagnostic and Statistical Manual of Mental Disorders, Fourth Edition (DSM-IV) and The International Statistical Classification of Diseases and Related Health Problems, Tenth Revision (ICD-10) are operationally based on symptoms and behavior. DSM-5 is scheduled for publication in 2013 (http://www.dsm5.org). The development of the upcoming version has been criticized, mainly for being overinclusive (most notably by Allen Frances, who was chair of the DSM-IV Task Force).[6] A lot of criticism has been published of the DSM system in general. Some have argued that mental disease is not biological but rather psychological or social. This meant denying physiological and biochemical aspects of depression. Others have acknowledged that depression can be a serious disease, but that it is overdiagnosed because of a less than optimal diagnostic system.[7]

The symptom-based psychiatric diagnostic systems are easy to understand and have contributed to expanding research and facilitating clinical communication. However, real individuals do not easily fit into diagnostic categories. Overemphasizing diagnosis may hinder the clinician trying to understand the patient within their full context, including disease origin and contributing factors. In 1999 Frances and Egger described psychiatry to be "where astronomy was before Copernicus and biology before Darwin."[8]

Despite their limitations, the DSM and ICD are still "used as diagnostic bibles by psychiatrists worldwide."[9] Insufficient diagnostic systems support psychiatrists treating syndromes instead of human beings. This does not mean that ongoing development of these systems will not be of some beneficial value.

However, diagnostic labels will seldom tell us about cause of a specific patient's depression, nor are they sufficient for comprehensive clinical judgment and determining suitable therapy. For good treatment the diagnostic formulation needs to be supplemented with patient history, blood and other physiological tests, psychological evaluation, and further investigations. Depression is a multifactorial disease. Winokur's paper, "All Roads Lead to Depression," emphasizes the many different factors for development of depression.[10] In research, interest has usually been focused on genetic, biomedical, psychological, and socioeconomic aspects of depression. The food we eat, our physical activity, circadian rhythm, working life, culture, and existential issues are areas less considered.

Comorbidity with Many Diseases

Depression is today a widespread disease that has a lot in common with other civilization and welfare diseases. People with depression often have other current somatic disease[11]. Comorbidity (existing along with another disease) for depression has been described for such specific diseases as cardiovascular disease, diabetes, multiple sclerosis, rheumatic and atopic diseases, some forms of cancer, and osteoporosis.[12] A possible relation between depression and metabolic syndrome or "civilization syndrome"[13] has also been discussed.[14] In these diseases depression is not only secondary to the somatic (physical) disease; it is often discovered prior to the somatic disease. Of course, depression is also a somatic disease with psychological aspects. Major depressive disorder has been described as a metabolic disorder in the form of "cerebral diabetes,"[15] "metabolic syndrome type II,"[16] or "metabolic encephalopathy."[17]. When comorbidity is strong it is reasonable to look for common origins and pathogenic mechanisms. Apart from genetic factors, inflammatory and immunologic mechanisms, autonomic nervous system impairment, oxidative stress as well as imbalances in insulin and glucose metabolism, cortisol and thyroid hormones play a role here.[18] Comorbidity is also an argument to look for treatment alternatives that address all of the patient's issues, both physical and psychological. In the same way that the general practitioner considers depression in patients with somatic manifestation, the psychiatrist ponders the somatic state of the patient.

Depression: Social, Individual, and Biochemical Perspectives

When a large proportion of people in a society suffer from depression, whether episodic or persistent, it is a social issue. As with other diseases, socioeconomic factors play a role. Even if depression is not the opposite of happiness, it has been claimed that people in the industrial world have become less happy, at least since the 1970s.[19] If we include all psychiatric illness, we are in a situation today where half the population, sometime during their life, will fulfill criteria for some psychiatric disease. This is partly explained by the change that has occurred in diagnostic methods. In Sweden between 1997 and 2003 we had an increase in number of people unable to work due to depression, burnout, and stress-related illness. Workplace changes are often pointed to as the main reason for this, but demanding changes, time-pressing limits, and new kinds of choices have been increasing in society in general. The accelerated pace of change may perhaps increase the rate of life experiences for a large part of the population. It is well-known that life events can be significant factors for depression.[20]

For the individual, depression means suffering. Studies show that the quality of life in patients suffering from medium or severe depressive states is compatible to what is found in serious somatic disease.

Depression is often regarded to be a psychological disorder that sometimes has somatic manifestations. Another view is that it is basically a biological disease that has psychological symptoms. Both of these concepts, however, are expressions of dualistic thinking. A more integrated perspective views the somatic and the mental symptoms as different aspects of the same disease.

Depression may be seen as an expression of unbalanced signal substances. Even if this is a partial mechanism, it is scarcely the original cause of the strong incidence for depression in our society today. Biochemical depression research has been preoccupied with serotonin and norepinephrine (noradrenalin) for over half a century, and most antidepressant drugs act on receptor sites for these two signal substances. But many other research findings also deserve attention. Many patients with depression have increased immunological parameters such as cytokines, which regulate inflammatory responses, supporting inflammation as part of the depression mechanism. Chronic low-grade inflammation is associated with altered tryptophan and tyrosine metabolism and this may contribute to psychiatric symptoms.[21] Other findings concern different hormone patterns, changed ratios between omega-6 and omega-3 polyunsaturated fatty acids, and low vitamin levels. Investigations of brain structure and function are also of great interest. We know too little about the primary changes that occur in depression. It is obvious that depression should not be seen only as a brain disorder. It has been pointed out that symptoms of somatic disease often precede the depressive feeling.[22]

NUTRITIONAL TREATMENT OF DEPRESSION
by Hugh D. Riordan, M.D.

Depression affects about 17 to 19 million American adults each year. It is possible to become depressed because of the lack of a sufficient amount of a single trace element. Did you know every medical text book, at least up until a few years ago, indicated that one of the most common effects of inadequate vitamin C is depression? We very seldom go to a psychiatrist who measures our vitamin C level.

Many years ago, I had a lady who was a teacher and she was profoundly depressed. She had three years of psychotherapy prior to coming to me. She had profound fatigue and was barely able to function at all. Our testing revealed she had no detectable vitamin C, so we gave her 500 milligrams of vitamin C a day—not very much by our standards.

In a couple of weeks, she thought a miracle had occurred. No miracle had occurred. She was low on vitamin C and depression is the natural consequence of that. She had very good insurance. A psychotherapist could have seen her every week for two years and the insurance company would have paid the entire bill. Our bill was for two office calls and three vitamin C levels. The company would not pay because vitamin C had nothing to do with depression, according to their payment schedule. If you are depressed, vitamin C is worth considering.

In studies at two area health care centers, 30 percent of new admissions with a diagnosis of depression had low plasma vitamin C levels. Actually, we did this study a number of years ago and found that if you took a hundred people who are depressed without checking their level and gave them all vitamin C, 30 percent would get better. Statistically that would be below the placebo level. That is why it is important to separate out the 30 percent from the large group, so the people who are low in vitamin C will obviously respond more to the vitamin C than the people who are not.

Of course, man and woman do not live by vitamin C alone. It is possible to become depressed because of the lack of a sufficient amount of a single trace element. The following is from an audio tape of a person who had this problem:

> I was getting more depressed. I had two grand babies coming at the end of July and I didn't want to see them. That's rather odd for a grandmother. I knew I wasn't up to helping my children with their children. I knew I had to teach. We needed the income. I never got any sleep and I wasn't worrying about my students. I teach learning disabled students. I love my job. I just didn't feel up to it and I knew something was wrong.
>
> I tried hypnosis to no avail. I tried several psychiatrists. I responded completely opposite of what the medication I took was supposed to do. This wasn't just a light depression. It was an inabil-

ity to cope with life, inability to enjoy my family. We couldn't go out to dinner because I was allergic to so many foods.

The thing that changed my life was persistence in letting them know that I wasn't feeling any better. They decided to give me double the amount of liquid zinc. Dr. Riordan told me how to take it. Instead of having it in a whole lot of water, I just had a smidgen of water. In two days' time when I had doubled the zinc, my husband said he had a new wife and he wasn't sure he could cope with me.

We even brought my daughter here who is severely depressed and we know she will get help. She has some of the same nutrient needs that I have but not the need for zinc. But we are all happy about the two new grandbabies. I have even been able to do better with my students.

There were several important points mentioned in that little piece. One point is to measure what's going on. If you gave zinc to 100 people who are depressed, 99 are not going to do much with that. In her case, zinc seemed to be her particular thing. It is very important to look at the individual biochemistry to see what is missing and what needs to be improved. Then you can do a great deal. She also indicated that she wasn't doing very well initially and that's why we have follow-up to see what's going on. Her initial zinc we knew was low and the initial amount we gave her was not sufficient to raise it to the level that she needed. Increasing her zinc was what eliminated her depression.

Keep in mind that zinc is involved in at least 100 enzyme systems in the brain alone. So, it's a very important trace mineral. Certainly not the only one, but one that is worthy of consideration when brain tissue function is not optimum.

Serotonin tends to improve mood and promote relaxation. If you're going to do a study on serotonin, you need to collect the urine for twenty-four hours. The lab will inform you that avocados, pineapple, eggplant, plums, walnuts, and pregnancy are going to affect the serotonin level.

According to a study done in Great Britain, 80 percent of people with mood disorders noticed that food choices affected how they felt. The food you choose [such as] avocados, bananas, and some walnuts, should pick up your serotonin level and, thus, enhance how you feel if you are depressed.

Sugar and alcohol are considered "mood stressors," according to a British study. In the same study, water, vegetables, fruit, and fish were considered "mood supporters." Actually, the researchers said water was number one for subjects wanting to improve how they felt. As we get older, one of the major problems is dehydration. When we were young, the ratio of water inside the cell to outside the cell is 1.2 to 1. There is more water inside the cell than there is outside. By the time we are sixty, the ratio is 0.8 to 1. Even if you are drinking enough water, you are dehydrating all the time. So the goal is to drink sufficient water.

The incidence of depressive disorders varies throughout the world. Japan has the lowest incidence of depression as does Korea—2 percent. Taiwan has 3 percent. The USA has 7 percent, New Zealand has 11 percent, and France has 16 percent. It would appear that the dietary choices people make have something to do with whether or not they are depressed. Japanese and Koreans eat fish. The omega-3 fat in most fish manipulates brain chemicals in ways that boost mood. You can, of course, measure fatty acids to see what levels you have. If the brain is not working well, feed it what it needs!

Most people don't appreciate that food has something to do with how they feel. In addition to general responses to various foods, adverse reactions to specific foods can lead to depression. I advocate using the cytotoxic test to detect adverse food reactions. This test is useful for people who have problems with brain fog or are not thinking well. The test is done by separating out the white cells and then mixing them with various food antigens. If the white blood cells are happy and healthy, that food is fine. If there's a kill off of white blood cells, then you have a positive cytotoxic test. Limiting cytotoxic foods can improve brain function.

Neurotransmitters are derived from amino acids, which can be measured in blood and urine. Abnormal amino acids can be corrected nutritionally which should improve neurotransmitter and brain function. Adequate amounts of fatty acids, which are in every cell membrane, can have a stabilizing effect on mood. The cells talk to each other through fatty acids in the membrane.

Inadequate thyroid function can lead to depression. One can measure a standard thyroid test, thyroid stimulating hormone (TSH), or thyroxine (T4). We measure triiodothyronine (T3), which is the active hormone that gets into the cell.

Hormonal changes, such as low testosterone, have been shown to affect depression. The same thing is true with female hormonal imbalances.

Short-term depression in response to unpleasant life events is normal and does not necessarily need an antidepressant. In our culture right now there is the notion that one should never feel depressed about anything. When certain things happen, you ought to feel depressed. If it is a short-term thing, it usually doesn't need treatment.

People who are depressed have been shown to breathe less deeply than people who are not depressed. You can de-stress by deep breathing. Take five deep breaths and hold each for six seconds. Do this four times a day. This decreases tension. You have two sides of the nervous system, the central nervous system and the autonomic nervous system. All day long we tense up with whatever is going on, and the autonomic nervous system tenses, too. It is like tightening a ratchet. When you take five deep breaths, it is like releasing the ratchet.

Exercise had been shown to be useful in eliminating depression. There are studies at the University of Wisconsin that show that getting people who are depressed to run in groups reduces the depression in about 85 percent of the people.

A psychologist said that we are all hit by the same hammer, so he made an interesting observation: "A person made three dolls: one of porcelain, one of plastic, one of steel. If you hit all three with a hammer, the porcelain would smash into pieces, the plastic one would be dented, and the steel doll would give off a musical note." So, it is not the hammer but how you are made that makes a difference.

Eat well, drink water, and check your nutrient levels and you will be like the doll made of steel.

(Used with permission of the Riordan Clinic, Wichita, KS
http://orthomolecular.org/library/articles/ocdepression.shtml)

IS DEPRESSION A DEFICIENCY DISEASE?

Depression and other psychiatric disorders are expressions of molecular imbalance in the brain. To some extent this may be affected by different nutrients in our food.[23] Studies have shown that brain function, and sometimes structure, is affected by food and stress. Many essential micronutrient deficiencies may lead to depression. Poor nutrient intake is based on badly balanced food, but the quality is also dependent on environmental pollution and acidification, preparation, and refinement of foods.

The quality of vegetarian foods may be worse than it once was. Some reports suggest that nutrient composition in fruits and vegetables have declined during the last century.[24] The quality of animal foods may likewise have become less nutritious.[25] The idea of modern foods being less nutritious has been questioned because the methods in different studies have changed over the decades, making comparisons uncertain. However, the precautionary principle tells us to seriously consider this possibility.

Perhaps depression is related to deficiencies of other environmental factors that *homo sapiens* evolved with and was adapted to. From an evolutionary perspective, man's current dissociation with nature is a fundamental issue. We have become disconnected from nature and all things natural. "Nature" is something we watch on television. In our society loneliness and alienation, and a lack of history and optimism about the future are expressions of human's loss of contact with self and nature. Thus, the question is if depression in a broader context is dependent on lack of nurture, nearness, and presence.

The term "nature-deficit disorder" was coined by Richard Louv, in describing exposure to nature as necessary for normal and healthy development of children.[26] He also emphasized the imperative that adults reconnect with nature.[27] We need to experience nature directly through our senses of sight, hearing, smell, taste, and feeling, rather than indirectly via television or computer interfaces.

Lack of medical drugs and psychotherapy is never the original cause for depression. Being familiar with depression research, I want to make it clear that no published science documents a primary deficiency of medical drugs or psychotherapy in humans. (Yes, there are exceptions, in which an individual was made dependent on medical drugs or non-professional psychotherapy.) In the best case, drugs and psychotherapy may be helpful as tools to assist the person in doing something about the origin of their depression.

Conventional Medical and Psychological Treatment Are Often Insufficient

After fifty years of antidepressant drug use the question is how important these have been for treatment of mood disorders.[28] It is often stated that two-thirds of patients improve at least fifty percent. In clinical practice of depression the results are often not as good. The placebo effect and other nonspecific effects are considerable in depression.[29] Patients often get wrong or insufficient drug treatment. Some percent become allergic to the drugs. Some cannot take these drugs for other medical reasons. Owing to side effects many patients also have a lower quality of life during long-term treatment. Many patients do not want to take drugs or end their treatment for different reasons. Eventually, roughly every second individual fulfilling current criteria for depression does not seek medical help.

In spite of all these objections, it is clear that antidepressant medications can be most helpful in deeper depressive states. It seems that antidepressants are better in more severe depressions, while the effectiveness for moderate or light depression is less supported in research studies.[30] Many patients with antidepressant treatment relapse, especially if they have not achieved full remission.[31] Antidepressant drugs can be effective in treatment of depressions, but are less beneficial in recurring depression or preventing relapse. It has been observed that antidepressants sometimes induce tolerance, withdrawal symptoms, or worsen long-time prognosis of recurrent depressive disorder.[32]

Cognitive (behavior) therapy and interpersonal therapy have documented effectiveness in the treatment of depression, and there is also some support for psychodynamic therapy. As with pharmacological treatment, psychotherapy is not appropriate for all patients. These treatments will not help some patients, and others do not want any kind of psychological treatment. When treatment with drugs or psychotherapy is finished, many patients will sooner or later relapse. Whatever treatment based on drugs or psychotherapy is given, it is pertinent to consider the origin and contributing mechanisms of the disease and whether the effects of treatment are directed at the symptoms, or the disease pathogenesis, or both. Antidepressant drugs have

some effects on the mechanisms of depression, but if the real causes
of the depression are untouched, the drug will only treat the symptoms. At the same time the use of drugs are indicated for many people
with depression, as it is an illness with strong suffering, risks, and
complications. Psychotherapy may treat psychosocial problems in the
patient's history, or at least have some learning value for the patient
to recognize their symptoms and risk factors for depression. But, often
the "talking cure" only has a symptomatic and short-term effect. What
is the benefit of symptomatic treatment of depression unless preventive
measures are also taken? Growing research supports that prevention
can be an option in decreasing depression.[33]

It's also clear that research on antidepressants and psychotherapy
has mostly been carried out with highly selected and motivated patient
groups that are not allowed to have other concurrent diseases. For this
reason the research results cannot be generalized for large numbers of
people with depression. The results of these selected patient groups
may be positive, but treatment results in clinical work with patients
are often just modest. This is even more the case if the patient has a
chronic or relapsing depression. Considering depressions in society,
the main prevention and treatment options available today are unsatisfactory. Thus, clinicians and researchers need to consider paths less
traveled in order to find more effective solutions.

Life Circumstances, Lifestyle, and Depression

People with depression often have unsatisfactory results from conventional treatments only. Many of those who initially benefit from acute
treatment relapse sooner or later. One possible explanation for this
is that treatments are not directed at the etiology, or cause, of their
depression. To improve treatment and prevention of depression, we
need to study and test changes of lifestyle and life circumstances. It
will be helpful to put depression in a broader context, and consider an
evolutionary perspective to find a more effective solution.

CHAPTER 2

AN EVOLUTIONARY VIEW
OF DEPRESSION

*"Nothing in biology makes sense except
in the light of evolution."*
—THEODOSIUS DOBZHANSKY (1900–1975)

In evolutionary perspective gives us an understanding for the origin and mechanisms of depression. This is important for developing effective prevention and treatment programs for depressive disorders.

SYSTEMS THINKING AND
EVOLUTIONARY MEDICINE

If you want to understand society and human social behavior you may study sociology. You will find that it has many aspects—you have to learn about history, culture, economy, geology, ecology, religion, politics, and psychology.[1] Similarly, if you want to learn about health and disease, you will need to acquire knowledge from physiology, biochemistry, ethology (animal behavior from a physiological, functional, and evolutionary perspective), different specialized medical disciplines, psychology, and other life sciences. For clinical work with individuals, you will have to integrate what is relevant in each specific case.

Systems theories, such as the biopsychosocial model[2] and systems biology,[3] emphasize holistic and interdisciplinary perspectives to understand health and disease relationships. By integrating such views with evolutionary aspects depression is seen in a different light. Considering biological, psychological, social, cultural, and evolutionary knowledge gives a richer understanding to depression. It is not enough to inquire about the history of a particular individual. We also need to know the history of our species.

Why Do We Get Sick?

Disease may develop when our genetically governed human needs—physiological, psychological, social, and existential—are not met. Nesse and Williams helped our understanding of disease origin using evolutionary theory.[4] Others gave explanations for psychiatric diseases in similar ways.[5] Depressions may be related to a need to avoid specific situations with threats, risks, high demands, and stress.[6] The way the human species lives today and our circumstances have also changed enormously in a comparatively short time. The implications of such rapid change should be considered when determining a cause for depression and other diseases.

Genetics and Environment— The Discordance Hypothesis

Eaton and his coworkers describe the discordance hypothesis in their book, *The Paleolithic Prescription.*[7] Its premise is that *homo sapiens* created our current environments and lifestyles during a relatively short period of time (a few thousand years). We have not adapted to these changes genetically, and this is the most important reason for the development of "civilization diseases." Our new environments and ways of living are a challenge to our inner healing mechanisms. The book focuses on somatic diseases such as coronary heart disease, hypertension, diabetes, chronic obstructive pulmonary disease, cancer, osteoporosis, caries, obesity, and alcohol related disease. This hypothesis has also been called the genome-lag hypothesis,[8] and was further developed for coronary heart disease,[9] type 2 diabetes,[10] and obesity.[11] In our view, the discordance hypothesis is important for the discussion of psychiatric disorder etiology, course, treatment, and prevention.

The concept that genes affect an individual's disposition for depression is of great interest. A combination of genetic susceptibility and specific life events increases the risk for depression.[12] As psychiatrist and researcher Robert Post commented, it is a shortcoming that a strong interest for molecular research is usually not combined with a simultaneous study of environmental factors.[13] When determining preventive action for depression it is important that gene research be integrated with the examination of lifestyle aspects, in the same way as it is for somatic disease.[14]

From Stone Age to Information Society

The oldest fossils of our own species, *homo sapiens,* are more than 150,000 years old.[15] The genetic changes that have occurred to humans since then are generally considered to be comparatively small. For millions of years our predecessors were hunter-gatherers. Ten thousand years ago agrarian communities with settled populations became more common. The industrial revolution evolved just two centuries ago, and the information society is only a generation old. Our life circumstances (something we as individuals cannot affect) and our lifestyles (which we as individuals or together with other people can change) are radically changing at an accelerated pace.

We have some limited knowledge about the prevalence for some somatic diseases over a few thousand years. However, we know very little about how common different psychiatric diseases were in the past. According to the documentation of some countries, the incidence of psychotic diseases (such as schizophrenia and bipolar disease) has increased during the recent 250 years.[16]

Let's take a look at our life today compared to what we believe it was like back in Stone Age:

COMPARATIVE ASPECTS OF HOMO SAPIENS' LIFE FROM AN EVOLUTIONARY PERSPECTIVE		
HUMAN LIFE FACTORS	PALEOLITHIC PERIOD	PRESENT TIME
Geographic spread	Living close to the equator, small seasonal variations	Living all over the earth, big seasonal variations
Time rhythm	Day and night equally long, only moonlight and starlight nightly, strong relation to moon phases	Day length variation during the year, electric light, shift work

Biosphere	Cleaner environment: air, water, earth	Contamination from chemicals, radioactive and electromagnetic radiation
Relationship to nature	Coexistence	Separation from nature, living inside houses
Community living form	Smaller and sparsely populated nomadic communities	Big cities with high living density
Social relations	Direct contact with fewer individuals	Less personal contact with masses, alienation, weak social capital
Human communication	Direct reciprocal contact in real life	Often one-direction in a virtual "time-room"
State of mind	Conscious here and now, mindfulness	Often flight from current to illusionary reality
Culture	Direct experience with few or no aids	Technically sophisticated "multimedia"
Nutrition	Unrefined animal (meat, fish, eggs) and vegetarian food	Recent 10,000 years: flour/read, milk/cheese, refined sugars and fats, alcohol, narcotics, drugs, smoking
Physical activity	Working with own strength	Using mechanic power, sedentary lifestyle
Technology	Simple working tools	Complicated technology, incomprehensible to the nonspecialist
Working life	Organized from needs of the closer group	Less clear relation to human needs, increased demands and time limits, less control
Economy	Barter, less individual possessions	Money economy, increasing e-business
Individual knowledge	Personal experience, oral tradition	Exponential growth of information, difficult to grasp as a whole

Daily Rhythm: Nature—Our Original Context

Man is part of nature. Like no other animal, humans change and destroy a large part of nature on earth.[17] Species of plants and animals are being exterminated before they are discovered.[18] The chemical pollution of nature affects us, with a large number of toxins being found in our cells. Smoking, alcohol, narcotics, and medical drugs contribute to the pollution of our bodies and through the cycle in nature of all environments. We live most of the time indoors, totally unlike our original circumstances.

Most people live far away from the geographic areas our ancestors inhabited near the equator. Living closer to the poles means greater seasonal light changes. This light variation may be the most important cause for seasonal depressions: seasonal affective disorder (SAD) has often been reported to be more common far away from the equator. However, these investigations are not unequivocal.[19]

ALCOHOLIC DEPRESSION

Abram Hoffer, M.D., Ph.D. writes:

My friend Bill W., [was] co-founder of Alcoholics Anonymous (Bill Wilson). We met in New York in 1960. Humphry Osmond and I introduced him to the concept of mega vitamin therapy. We described the results we had seen with our schizophrenic patients, some of whom were also alcoholic. We also told him about its many other properties. It was therapeutic for arthritis, for some cases of senility and it lowered cholesterol levels.

Bill was very curious about it and began to take niacin, 3 g [grams] daily. Within a few weeks fatigue and depression which had plagued him for years were gone. He gave it to 30 of his close friends in AA and persuaded them to try it. Within 6 months he was convinced that it would be very helpful to alcoholics. Of the thirty, 10 were free of anxiety, tension and depression in one month. Another 10 were well in two months. He decided that the chemical or medical terms for this vitamin were not appropriate. He wanted to persuade members of AA, especially the doctors in AA, that this would be a useful addition to treatment and he needed a term that could be more readily popularized. He asked me the names that had been used. I told him it was originally known as vitamin B$_3$. This was the term Bill wanted. In his first report to physicians in AA he called it "The Vitamin B$_3$ Therapy." Thousands of copies of this extraordinary pamphlet were distributed. Eventually the name came back and today even the most conservative medical journals are using the term vitamin B$_3$.

Bill became unpopular with the members of the board of AA International. The medical members who had been appointed by Bill, felt that he had no business messing about with treatment using vitamins. They also "knew" vitamin B$_3$ could not be therapeutic as Bill had found it to be. For this reason Bill provided information to the medical members of AA outside of the National Board, distributing two of his amazing pamphlets. They are now not readily available. [Their contents are summarized in *The Vitamin Cure for Alcoholism*, by A. Hoffer and A. W. Saul.]

—Excerpt from *Vitamin B$_3$: Niacin and Its Amide*,
http://www.doctoryourself.com/hoffer_niacin.html

Dr. Hoffer continues:

Ever since I met Bill W., the cofounder of Alcoholics Anonymous and we became close friends, I have had a personal interest in the treatment of alcoholism. Bill taught that there were three components to the treatment of alcoholism: spiritual, mental, and medical. AA provided a spiritual home for alcoholics that many could not find anywhere else and helped them sustain abstinence. But for many AA alone was not enough; not everyone in AA had achieved a comfortable sobriety. Bill recognized that the other two components were important. When he heard of our use of niacin for treating alcoholics, he became very enthusiastic about it because niacin gave these unfortunate patients immense relief from their chronic depression and other physical and mental complaints. Nutritional factors have been shown to be very successful on treating this condition. When alcoholics are able to abstain on their own, this is the way to go. Some of them can even become social drinkers on a very small scale. I have not found many who could. But I think that if started on the program very early, many more could achieve normalcy. I know of many alcoholics who did not want to stop drinking, but did agree to take niacin. Over the years, they gradually were able to reduce their intake until they brought it under control. I suspect that treatment centers using those ideas will be made available one day, and will be much more successful than the standard treatment today. This all too often still consists of dumping them into hospitals and letting them dry out, with severe pain and suffering. When they are discharged, most go right back to the alcohol, the most dangerous and widely used street drug available without a prescription.

—Excerpt from the introduction to *A Protocol for Alcohol,* http://www.doctoryourself. com/alcoholism.html

Our daily rhythm is governed by genes in every cell. The twenty-four-hour circadian rhythm is repeatedly found among almost all animals and even among most plants. It has been shown that disruption of circadian clocks affects metabolism, brain function, and behavior in mice.[20] It is natural for humans to sleep in darkness, and we feel at our best when we alternate between work, activity, rest, and recreation. Important physiologic processes are going on during sleep. Long-time poor sleep disturbs carbohydrate metabolism and endocrine functions.[21] This may increase risk for cardiovascular disease, type 2 diabetes, and obesity. Poor sleep may also be a risk factor for or an early symptom of depression. In our current twenty-four-hour society our daily rhythm is governed not only by the celestial bodies, but to a great extent by the sources of light created by man. Sleep supporting actions are important in depression treatment and prevention.

It's a common view that a close contact with nature has a beneficial effect on depression, positively affecting our mental well-being as well as improving the prognosis for some physical diseases.[23] Very little depression research has been carried out on this. Single studies have shown that walking and outdoor physical activity have an antidepressant effect. The environment in natural areas and in urban built-up areas differs in many ways. In a natural setting air contains more negative ions. In a small study of a group of patients with seasonal affective disorder (SAD) the group given high-dose negative ions had a significantly better antidepressant effect compared to those receiving low-dose negative ions.[24] In a later study the treatment group with SAD was given light therapy. Two control groups were treated with negative ions in different concentrations. Those receiving light ther-

SLEEP PROBLEMS

"Sleep my little baby.
Sleep until the morning.
Sleep until the sunrise,
At the new days dawning."
—TRADITIONAL SPANISH LULLABY

Disturbed sleep may be the first symptom experienced by lots of people with different diseases. In depression it is common to have various sleeping problems, such as difficulty in falling asleep, having interrupted sleep, or waking up early. Some of us sleep too little, others too much. It is especially valuable to be able to go into the deep sleep stage, as it is essential for memory function and production of sex and growth hormones with anabolic effects. Sleeping well is much easier when our inner and outer environment is in a harmonious state—when we are not overly disturbed by inner tension, worry, and anxiety, nor by light, noise, or other outer stimuli. The importance of sleep to our health is described in *Lights Out: Sleep, Sugar, and Survival,* by T. S. Wiley.[22]

apy and those with a higher concentration of negative ions reported a significant antidepressant effect compared to the low-dose group.[25] The mechanism for the effect of ions is unclear, but negative ions are more abundant in natural settings. This may be one reason why it feels good to be close to waters and forests.

Being outdoors regularly and having good lighting and nearness to windows while indoors may lessen the risk for SAD.[26] There is limited research supporting the theory that walking outdoors may be as helpful as light therapy in treating SAD.[27] However, there are certainly many factors active in this treatment: light, temperature, movement, activity, and outdoor nature experience. In one study, walking combined with a multivitamin preparation gave a positive effect for women with depression.[28]

FOOD: WE ARE WHAT WE EAT

Hunter-gatherers have eaten animal and vegetarian food in different proportions. In the industrial world at least two-thirds of our food is refined, and was unknown to a Stone Age dweller. The current change of food in the developing world could be the biggest medical experiment ever, although unethical, unscientific, and uncontrolled.[29] This may be important not only for cardiovascular disease, diabetes, and obesity,[30] but also for mental disease.[31]

Nutrition is given very little attention in the educations of physicians and nursing staff. So, quite naturally, it is not considered important in clinical work either. This is strange, considering the enormous importance of nutrition actually substantiated by research. Human molecules, cells, and organs are built from what we eat. The structure, functions, and energy of our bodies are based on nutrition. Why is there such a strong resistance to incorporate this knowledge into traditional medicine? David Horrobin (1939–2003) discussed this in a paper published shortly after his untimely death. The different arguments for not applying modern nutrition knowledge are listed below, according to his article.[32]

Reductionist scientist	Conservative research attitude within current paradigm. We know too little and can only study one variable at a time. Trial program will last the lifetime of many researchers.
Nutritionist/ dietitian	The solution is to educate people to eat a properly varied diet with several portions of fruits and vegetables each day.
Drug-oriented regulator	Every ingredient must meet full pharmaceutical good manufacturing practice (GMP) standards and tolerance limits to be licensed for therapeutic purposes and make medicinal claims.
Pharmaceutical company	No interest in products that cannot be given patent protection.
Government	No interest to address a need not worthwhile for private enterprise in a free-market society.

This list shows that the resistance to nutrition knowledge within medicine is dependent on lack of knowledge, tradition, greed, and fear of losing money and power. Excluding lifestyle factors helps maintain this position, since nutrition and other treatments aimed at the causes for illness may undermine the current industry, which profits from chronic illness.

Omega-3 Fatty Acids

In a Norwegian qualitative study, students, nurses, and psychiatrists were interviewed about the effect of omega-3 fats on depression.[33] It was found that (1) nutrition was considered important, but few evaluations of nutritional status, need, or effects were made; (2) the knowledge of effects from omega-3 was lacking; and (3) there was an unclear division among the health personnel concerning responsibility for nutrition aspects.

The message has often been that treatment of disease implies medication and scalpel, while nutritional contents and physical activity are of minor importance. This view is still common within psychiatry, which continues the dualistic division of an individual into body and soul. In psychiatry it's been uncommon to ask the patient about food intake, physical activity, and other lifestyle aspects. Modern neuroradiologic investigations studying brain structure and function may help change this. Supplementing polyunsaturated fatty acids may change the brain structure in rats[34] and humans.[35] Dietary fish oil increased dopamine levels in the frontal cortex of rat brain.[36]

People who are depressed often eat less protein and may consume more fast carbohydrates. The foods of our time, together with physical inactivity and stress, may be the most important cause of metabolic syndrome, a collection of heart disease risk factors, and its related diseases. Modern food usually means a smaller consumption of omega-3 fatty acids compared to consumption of omega-6. We need these fats in well-balanced amounts as necessary components of the cell membranes in the nervous system and the rest of the body. The essential omega-3 fatty acids EPA and DHA are most abundant in fatty fish, commonly found in the cold waters on earth. A negative correlation has been found between fish consumption and the prevalence of depression in different countries.[37] Supplementing EPA in patients who did not respond to antidepressant drugs resulted in faster recovery compared to patients treated with placebo.[38] Fish oil with EPA/DHA in a two-to-one ratio also gave significant positive effect,[39] while treatment with DHA only gave mixed results.[40]

Sugar

Refined sugar intake is very high today. Sugar dependency is often discussed in mass media. This dependency has been shown in animal studies.[41] One study, covering six countries, described a high correlation between sugar consumption and depression.[42] There are a lot of case studies in popular literature describing that people who remove refined sugar from their diet feel better and may recover from depres-

SUGAR BLUES

As the well-known song goes, "I got those sugar blues." Most people like sweet foods from birth. Certainly, we can understand there are evolutionary aspects to this. The positive effect of sucrose is, however, very short. Lots of people have a tendency to get addicted to sugar and sweeteners. This partly depends on our genetic make-up. Sugar may be the first addiction for people who develop other substance addictions later on.

Our culture is sugar contaminated, and the dark side of sugar consumption is related to its specific effects in the body. It is not only your teeth that suffer. Glucose competes with vitamin C, and a high sugar intake disturbs nutritional balance leading to vitamin and mineral depletion. Furthermore, sugar drives insulin and promotes inflammatory mechanisms, which may contribute to all sorts of diseases. Sugar increases the risk for development of cardiovascular disease, diabetes, obesity, and cancer, as well as depression and anxiety. These effects have been described in books like *The Saccharine Disease* by Thomas L. Cleave, and *Sugar Blues* by William Dufty.[44] (A curious side note: Dufty learned about the dangers of sugar from the famous film actress Gloria Swanson, whom he later married.)

sion and other diseases. It is well known that sugar has a very short positive mental effect. People with or without depression often take sugar as a short-term stimulant, but many find that it is the beginning of a vicious cycle resulting in symptoms like fatigue, irritability, insomnia, and mood degeneration. Larry Christensen described that some patients with fatigue and other depressive symptoms recovered when sucrose and caffeine were eliminated. In one single-blind randomized study depressive patients got significantly better than the control group three weeks after they excluded sucrose and caffeine from their diet.[43]

Nutritional Deficiency and Depression

Deficiencies of several essential nutrients are found also in industrial countries. Especially prone to this are groups that usually do not use nutritional supplements.[45] People under stress may have higher needs for certain nutrients. Food choices vary considerably among young people. The increase of poor mental health in youth in the industrial world after World War II may have many reasons, including nutritional deficiency. In a study of teens in the United States a correlation was found between unbalanced food intake and dysthymia (chronic low-level depression) and suicidal symptoms, while other socioeconomic factors had no relation.[46] Studies point to folic acid[47] and other B vitamins, vitamin C,[48] vitamin D,[49] selenium,[50] magnesium,[51] zinc,[52] and chromium[53] as being of interest in depression treatment. Of course, the total nutrient balance is important, as well as our own biochemical individuality. Ecological (natural) food, vegetarian as well as animal, may be more nutritious than "modern" conventional food.

PHYSICAL ACTIVITY

An athletic, bodybuilding confidant of mine would not even listen to me (AWS) on the phone until I went out and ran a couple of miles. Exercise is a known antidepressant. Studies with mice show that running is a crucial factor for brain neurogenesis.[54] Native peoples often, but not always, had a physical strength and condition comparable to the most physically active in our current society.[55] A minority of people in industrial societies have a strong physique, owing to their profession or physical training. A sedentary life with inactivity and passivity may contribute to depression. Inactivity, in a broad meaning, is a cardinal symptom of depression. Research also supports the hypothesis that lower levels of physical activity in childhood and adolescence may be a risk factor for adult depression.[56]

People with a higher level of physical activity have fewer symptoms of depression. Good physical condition and strength have a preventive effect on depression.[57] Physical training is a good complement to conventional treatment for depression, but knowledge about using it systematically for this purpose is still lacking in health care. In a controlled study of patients with major depression, a group participating in physical training three times a week was compared to antidepressant drug treatment. One group was treated with physical training, another received sertraline, and a third group was treated with both options. After eight weeks the two groups with the drug had a better effect than the group receiving only physical training. After sixteen weeks all three groups had a similar effect.[58] In a follow-up six months later, the group

WHY EXERCISE?

*"The nervous system and the muscles need exercise
in order that their vital metamorphoses shall
contribute to the normal chemical composition of
the blood that bathes the brain."*
—WILLIAM JAMES (1842–1910)

We all know that moderate physical training is good. It must be applied to our individual resources. Several models describing why physical activity is good for our mental health have been proposed. The anthropological hypothesis point to our history as hunters and gatherers. The temperature hypothesis states that intensive training increases body temperature, benefitting our state of mind. Biochemical theories describe increased tissue concentrations of endorphins, serotonin, and norepinephrine, while psychological hypotheses emphasize that increased self-control and distraction are important.

given only physical training had a better result than the other groups.[59] An explanation for this is that the group not receiving the drug knew that the physical training had helped them, and had continued it on their own. They were in charge of their own treatment.

It is reasonable that physical activity strengthens self-experience and lessens risk of relapse. Physical activity stimulates a lot of physiologic functions such as hormones and signal substances. Many studies in this area are of less than optimal quality,[60] but even if evidence is minimal, it does not mean that physical activity should be neglected. Instead it should be studied as a complementary technique in the treatment and prevention of depression.

SOCIAL SITUATION AND DEPRESSION

Hunter-gatherers lived in small, sometimes nomadic groups. Today we commonly live in cities with lots of people, with whom we have mainly anonymous contact. You may meet more persons in a day than Stone Age humans encountered during a lifetime. Pictures of and our ideas of other humans affect us profoundly, and modern humans are subject to extensive and rapid sensory impressions that have no ancient counterpart, potentially creating a subconscious, mental overload.

Stone Age societies were less hierarchic than modern societies. Studies of native people have supported the theory that decisions may have been made in a more anarchistic, democratic way.[61] Hierarchy and increased inequality came into existence with the growth of agricultural communities. The occurrence of many diseases increased as larger groups of people settled together, and when food evolved into milk and bread.[62] The advent of industrial society, irrespective of its blessings, further removed us from our origins with an increasingly altered environment, unnatural food, physical inactivity, and stress. Our communities became more complex. To a certain extent we adapted to living in towns, and we may like it,[63] but this lifestyle is not without drawbacks. Inequalities have increased within and between many countries in recent times. Even if emergency medicine has been successful, with lower infant mortality and longer life expectancy, the burden of illness is enormous today. To a large extent it is related to social conditions and modern lifestyles. Globalization affects human cultures thoroughly and can be a factor negatively affecting mental health.[64]

Depression is reported to be more common in urban communities compared to rural areas,[65] and is also more common among people with poorer socioeconomic conditions. Why these situations are related to more physical and mental illness is not fully known. It may be related not only to economic and psychosocial factors, but also to mediating factors as poor nutrition, physical inactivity, and sleeping problems. The real mechanisms need more investigation so programs for treatment and prevention can be developed.

The Value of Work

Work has central meaning to humans. During Stone Age the working process was comprehensive, varied, and gave immediate yield. The work carried out had developed and adapted over thousands of years. Among many native people working time was shorter compared to our current "efficient" society. Stress was acute, transient, and had a clearly defined source. We are programmed to manage that kind

STRAIGHTENING OUT DEPRESSION

Spinal manipulation may help relieve depression. Does back pain and muscle tension cause depression, or does depression cause muscle tension and back pain? This chicken-or-the-egg argument may be resolved by a therapeutic trial of chiropractic adjustment. Although I (AWS) taught clinical nutrition at a chiropractic college, I am not a chiropractor. Still, some things rubbed off on me from working with a lot of chiropractors and chiropractic students. You might like to look up these case studies:

Mahanidis, T. "Improvement in Quality of Life in a Patient with Depression Undergoing Chiropractic Care Using Torque Release Technique: A Case Study." *J Vertebral Subluxation Research* (Jan 31, 2010).

Desaulniers, A. M. J. "Effect of Subluxation-Based Chiropractic Care on Quality of Life in a Patient With Major Depression." *J Vertebral Subluxation Research* (Apr 23, 2008).

of stress and to respond quickly by fighting, fleeing, or playing dead. In chronic stress situations, which are more common today, we are unable to resolve problems with such immediate responses. In this case, stress can develop into depression.

In the industrial and informational societies of today, communities are intimately tied to technology. Our work is often divided into different specializations and types of work we did not have in the past and have not adapted to over a long period of time. Most people do not see and are not involved in the entire process of the work they do, and never see its full context or eventual outcome. Compensation for the work they do is usually delayed in time.

Modern information technology (IT) has become advanced and ubiquitous, and is often incomprehensible rather than user friendly. In worst cases, technology can substitute for our own experience and judgment. IT gives us new positive options, but also the risk for escapism, abuse, and depression.[66]

Over the past few decades computer technology has had a tremendous impact in speeding up work expectations, as well as in society as a whole.[67] The increased stress experienced as a result raises stress hormones and related ill-health. Depression can thus be connected to unemployment, reorganization, and the modern working environment.[68] A healthy working life should decrease some of the burden of depression.

Among early native societies, biological relatives often lived close to each other and parents were usually near to their small children. Family structures and social patterns varied considerably, but roles and expectations were clear. Natural rhythms were important for a sense of meaning and the development of culture and religion in prehistoric societies. Play, rituals, and creativity were important forms of expression among early people, just as they are for modern people.[69] Unfortunately, the areas in which we can integrate play and creativity have been reduced in contemporary society, partly replaced by superficial mass culture. Spectator sports and games often lead to passivity and escapism. Creative ability is a common characteristic among people with depression, but this ability may be reduced during depression. Providing stimulating options for creativity may also help in healing mood disorder.

The monotheistic world religions that evolved in agricultural settings provided an ethical code for building complicated societies.[70] A couple of generations ago, religion and family unity were important and provided strict standards and values. Today we get the impression that we have many choices. However, research has found that participants with more choices actually performed and felt worse than those who did not have such options.[71] When choices are illusionary, it leads to frustration. Increased depression during the last century has been attributed to less religiousness in industrial societies. The decrease of religious power is a form of freedom, but existential questions can become more difficult and feelings of loss and emptiness may grow.

Stress Management

Contemporary society imposes a lot of stress on our Stone Age genes. A healthy lifestyle more in sync with our biological heritage is optimal to manage stress. We also have inborn abilities to cope with the stresses of life that challenged our ancestors long ago.

POSTURAL PRESENTATION

One counselor friend of mine (AWS) not only carefully listens; he carefully observes how a client is sitting. When a client is miserable, he deliberately makes the person change how they are sitting. The counselor requires them to rearrange their posture, sit up straighter, uncross a crossed leg, shift a shoulder, turn their head, pivot on a hip. It may work as a pattern interrupt: it seems to indeed help mood and costs nothing to try.

This is reminiscent of that strict old school teacher who would not let you slouch, the finishing school that made young ladies walk around with a book atop their head to make them stand up straight, or the military drill instructor who constantly bellowed "Attention!" It is harder to be depressed when you are focused on a physical task. Moving itself is distracting: try two hours of square dancing or doing the polka and see how depressed you feel. Afterwards, you may want to sit down, but you certainly will not *feel* down.

Conventional Treatment and/or Lifestyle Change

The following list shows just a few examples of environment and life-style changes that have occurred over comparatively few generations, which may affect health and possibly also the incidence and course of depressions:

1. Refined sugars have become a significant part of a nutrient-depleted diet.

2. Industrialization of food production has disrupted the quality of both animal and vegetarian foods.

3. We have been exposed to thousands of man-made chemicals invented in the last century.

4. We now live mostly indoors, and get less physical activity, less sunshine, and more contact with electromagnetic fields.

5. Stress in society has increased, with fewer natural recovery periods.

We need new approaches if we want to successfully attack the depression epidemic and have a vision of a healthier civilization. Methods that focus on improving life conditions and lifestyle choices have great potential for long-term treatment and prevention. Studies of somatic disease—heart disease, type 2 diabetes, obesity, and many forms of cancer—have shown that lifestyle change can be at least as good as the best drugs for treating these diseases.[72]

It has been claimed that considering lifestyle factors is of no value in depression treatment. These factors were deemed so unimportant that they were ignored and not taken into account or controlled in research. Thus, scientific knowledge of the impact of lifestyle on depression is quite limited.[73] But the time is ripe for many exciting questions in this field. From a holistic view, new research should develop that includes the evolutionary aspects of depression. Research methodologies need to recognize that lifestyle factors and drugs cannot be investigated in the same way. Combined treatments should also be studied, because depression is often multifactorial. The costs to the individual and society, side effects, and other life factors are important areas to consider.

There is much to gain in including nutrition, physical activity, and stress management in psychiatric evaluation, treatment, and guidelines. Research in psychology, physiology, and biochemistry needs to be integrated with detailed clinical work to fully understand the role of lifestyle in the pathogenesis and treatment of depression.

The development of lifestyle treatment for depression may be considered not "cost-effective," but when these methods are shown to be both effective and safe, individuals—and society as a whole—will be very interested in them. It is also significant that these same treatments can help with metabolic disease and other civilization diseases. These therapeutic measures work in harmony with our genetic heritage and human community development. Furthermore, people ask for complementary forms of treatment,[74] so they are positively inclined toward them.

Working with lifestyle makes it easier to adopt a health perspective instead of a disease view. A growing field in psychology is working with enhancing well-being and ameliorating depressive symptoms. A meta-analysis of positive psychological interventions, including cognitive and behavior strategies, supports the development of these methods for depression treatment.[75] A prospective study of 5,566 people showed that those with low positive well-being were seven times more likely to be depressed ten years after treatment.[76]

Still, it is not easy for an individual to change his or her lifestyle. Let us remember that this question is not only personal, but also social and political. Nutrition, physical and mental activity, daily rhythm, stress, and other behaviors are affected by political, economic, commercial, and cultural interests. Authorities, health care, politicians, researchers, and other interested people have a huge responsibility to share and develop knowledge, laws, and guidelines that make it possible for us to live in harmony with our biological, psychological, social, and existential prerequisites.

CHAPTER 3

CONVENTIONAL TREATMENT AND TRADITIONAL SCIENCE

"There is a principle which is a bar against all information, which is proof against all arguments, and which cannot fail to keep man in everlasting ignorance. That principle is contempt prior to investigation."

—WILLIAM PALEY (1743–1805), OFTEN ATTRIBUTED TO HERBERT SPENCER (1820–1903)

In the United States 11 percent of the population are on antidepressants, and their use has increased by 400 percent in fifteen years. Among classes of medication these drugs are the third most prescribed, but the first in the eighteen to forty-four age group.[1] Medical drugs today are developed for populations instead of individuals. The reason is that pharmaceutical drugs are big business with powerful global interests.

CONVENTIONAL TREATMENTS FOR DEPRESSION

Current treatment of depression is mainly directed at symptoms, and the foremost instruments for treatment are antidepressant drugs and psychotherapy. Often these methods are described as the best available. For a lot of people this treatment is very important and sometimes even lifesaving. It is commonly discussed which of these methods is best for depression treatment. A combination of medication and psychotherapy is often helpful for the individual. Antidepressants and psychotherapeutic methods will certainly be further advanced, but it should be noted that the potential for treatment that focuses on symptoms is limited. Too often these treatments are insufficient and side effects are common. There is some evidence that patients can develop tolerance to antidepressants.[2] The most common idea explaining the neurochemistry of depression has been that it is caused by an impairment of the monoamine neurotransmitters (serotonin, norepinephrine, and dopamine). However, another position is that homeostasis of monoamines is actually functioning properly in most patients with depression. It has been suggested that chronic drug exposure leads to *oppositional tolerance,* where the brain compensates for the antidepressants in an attempt to recover its normal processes. This may explain why discontinuation of antidepressant drugs can increase the risk for relapse.[3]

Electroconvulsive Therapy

Electroconvulsive therapy (ECT) can be a treatment for the most difficult depressions. The mechanisms for this treatment are still debated. Normalization of neuroendocrine dysfunction is usually seen as the most probable explanation.[4] Short-term memory problems are quite common in ECT. That the treatment may lead to less common long-term cognitive problems has been questioned, and is now recognized.[5] Vitamin B_1 has been suggested to prevent cognitive problems related to ECT.[6] This had already been reported by Gould in the early 1950s. He used a combination of vitamins B_1, B_2, B_3, B_5, B_6, and C given parenterally (via infusion or injection) before ECT and observed that memory impairment was reduced or absent.[7] Abram Hoffer also reported good results with niacin to prevent confusion after ECT.

Psychopharmacology

Current psychopharmacology has mostly been directed at monoamine receptor inhibition or stimulation. This may change, as other depression hypotheses have been developed.[8] Orthomolecular medicine has been interested in using nutrients as metabolic precursors. These are the molecules used in the biochemical processes of metabolism, including receptor interaction. Several vitamins and minerals participate in cofactors or coenzymes, which are necessary for thousands of biochemical reactions in the body. Nutrients also modulate gene expression.[9] All of these can therefore be significant factors for the physical causes of depression.

MAKING SENSE OF SCIENCE

"When an old and distinguished person speaks to you, listen to him carefully and with respect—but do not believe him. Never put your trust into anything but your own intellect. Your elder, no matter whether he has grey hair or has lost his hair, no matter whether he is a Nobel laureate, may be wrong. The world progresses, year by year, century by century, as the members of the younger generation find out what was wrong among the things that their elders said. So you must always be skeptical—always think for yourself."

—LINUS PAULING (1901–1994)

Good science means careful observation, hypothesis formulation and testing, theory building, and replication of experiments. In the development of science, curiosity, persistence, critical—including self-critical—thinking, openness, honesty, respect, and humbleness have been important and necessary characteristics. To acquire knowledge it is important to think for yourself, not only inside the box, but also outside the box. Good science is about studying reality and from that drawing a map.

Bad science is different. Opinion is considered as fact. Generalizing is done from single observations. Personal reviews and consensus are overemphasized. Meta-analyses are considered more important than direct observation. Double-blind methodology is praised even when it is not applicable. Bad science is often dependent on commercial, political, and ideological interests. And when test results are undesirable they are withheld and not published. In bad science you keep faith with the map instead of investigating and reporting reality.

The application of scientific standards of proof in medicine is not easy and is often biased.[10] A large part of the conventional medical research published in well-known journals is serious good science. However, there are also a lot of published papers of low quality due to their poor research methodology. Medicine has naturally changed a lot during the last century, but it may be a problem that basic knowledge of physiology and biochemistry has often been de-emphasized because of isolated but highly publicized accomplishments in molecular and genetic research.[11]

A big problem is the way science is treated outside of the scientific literature. In mainstream media the word "science" is often used in a careless, manipulating, and fraudulent manner.

Randomized Controlled Trials (RCT)

The randomized controlled trial (RCT) is considered "the gold standard" for the study of medical drugs. This is based on the assumption that patients can be rationally characterized and compared in similar groups. There are many reasons why this is no easy task. We are all biochemically different, and recognizing this is essential to successfully determine what treatment may help the individual. There may be important factors that are not controlled for in the study parameters. An RCT is usually blinded to prevent participants from knowing which treatment is applied, but patients may find out in intervention studies. This information can affect the experience, healing process, and self-rating. Also, clinicians treat individuals, not diagnoses. The statistically defined participant in research is always different from a real person. The clinical consultation situation is different from the research-controlled patient consultation.

In some medical disciplines it is recognized that the RCT is not always the best research method, and in fact over-reliance on this model is not scientifically sound.[12]

In psychiatry the study sample participants in the RCT are often not representative for the target population of clinical patient groups. The vast majority of depression patients who are appropriate for clinical treatment do not pass common exclusion criteria for antidepressant clinical trials.[13] Still, most of these patients are judged by the clinician to potentially benefit from antidepressant treatment. It is important to realize that the goal of the pharmaceutical industry is to demonstrate good outcome in time- and cost-effective efficacy trials. For the doctor the aim is to apply evidence-based medicine (EBM) to real-world patients. These two goals are very different and imply a conflict both in clinical practice and research. Also, the recruitment of representative patient samples poses a complex and difficult process in psychotherapy research, and this may compromise the evidence value of these trials.[14]

In clinical drug trials the main outcome measure has been significant differences on rating scales between groups. However, most important is how many patients achieve a clinically meaningful response. Such an analysis focuses more on the individual patient.[15]

Professor John Ioannidis at Tufts University in Boston has pointed out that most published research findings are false.[16] He explains this is because of problems both with the design of the trials and the interpretation of their results.

Is the Use of Placebos Scientific?

Placebos have been used for centuries. In the 1950s, a classic work by Henry K. Beecher reported that the therapeutic effect of placebos on patients was quite powerful.[17] Forty years later, a re-analysis of the same trials strongly questioned this, and the authors pointed out that "the placebo topic seems to invite sloppy methodological thinking."[18] While the value of RCTs and placebos has been upheld in psychiatric circles for a long time, "the scientific integrity of RCTs themselves has been corrupted in the hands of the pharmaceutical industry."[19] One example of their unscientific aspects is the fact that the contents of placebo pills are often not reported.[20]

Abram Hoffer conducted some of the first double-blind placebo-controlled studies in the history of psychiatry.[21] When he saw the way double-blind methodology was used by others some years later he became an early critic of studies in which placebos are just one of many scientific methodologies.[22] In a way, the double-blind methodology is based on lying to the patient, which is different from the casual clinical situation. This may be agreed to as part of the study, but our point is that it also devalues such research trials. The fact is that patients are not that dumb. They will be interested to know which treatment they get, and they will often find out what group they belong to. If they suspect they are getting placebo treatment they may add other treatments themselves. Some fields have also long recognized that the double-blind methodology may be unethically applied.[23]

Meta-Analyses

A meta-analysis takes the results from different, independent studies on a topic and combines their findings to try to identify common patterns. Meta-analyses may have some value if they are used wisely as part of a systematic review. However, meta-analyses are often used in inappropriate ways.[24] It is common knowledge that the cardinal rules for using this advanced method are broken, and it is especially common that the included analyses are unrelated and inappropriate for comparison. This is the case with some meta-analyses where a varied intake of antioxidant supplements, other nutrients, and drugs were used in quite diverse populations of both sick and healthy people.[25] The conclusions from these studies were mostly negative toward nutrient treatment. Bjelakovic's 2007 study on this topic in *The Journal of the American Medical Association (JAMA)* was critically analyzed for its poor methodology.[26] Later, when the study was re-analyzed with a more appropriate methodology, it actually supported an integrated approach using nutrients in a sound way.[27]

It has been shown that meta-analyses of published clinical trials overestimate the effect magnitude of antidepressant drugs. One reason is that publication and reporting has been selective. If unpublished data submitted to the drug regulatory authorities is included, the results are further diminished.[28]

Consensus

There is a strong tendency for consensus in medicine. The well-known author and filmmaker Michael Crichton (1942–2008), who was educated as an M.D., wrote: "Let's be clear: the work of science has nothing whatever to do with consensus. Consensus is the business of politics. Science, on the contrary, requires only one investigator who happens to be right, which means that he or she has results that are verifiable by reference to the real world. In science consensus is irrelevant. What is relevant is reproducible results. The greatest scientists in history are great precisely because they broke with the consensus. There is no such thing as consensus science. If it's consensus, it isn't science. If it's science, it isn't consensus. Period."

Peer-Review

The peer-review system has some validity in helping scientists improve their articles. However, it has too often inhibited publication of scientific findings, or hypotheses, which were unconventional.[29]

Ghostwriting

Time and again scientific misconduct is reported.[30] A phenomenon revealed during recent years is that pharmaceutical companies have systematically been involved in ghostwriting articles for medical scientific journals.[31] This means that the text was first written by people in the company, but more respected scientists within the field were paid as authors even if they had a negligible or no role in the reported studies. The purpose of such fabricated disinformation is primarily to increase sales of products that obviously are not good enough themselves. But it also sponsors the overvaluation of belief in xenobiotic (sometimes called toximolecular) drugs as opposed to cheaper natural treatments. One problem is a reliance on review papers: these publications often use secondary sources instead of primary sources. Another factor is the failure of the physicians who endorsed the ghostwritten work to acknowledge that they received industry support. Medical ghostwriting threatens public health, and medical centers should prohibit it as "academic misconduct akin to plagiarism or falsifying data."[32]

The occurrence of inappropriate (honorary and ghost) authors has been recognized more in recent years. It seems that in at least six high-impact medical journals this kind of authorship has decreased from 29.1 percent in 1996 to 21.0 percent in 2008.[33] Still, inappropriate authorship remains a problem in these supposedly reputable medical journals.

Is Science More Business, Ideology, or Religion?

Modern science is big business.[34] Medical science has also become more dependent on money; it's a money-based medicine. The fusion between universities and industry has resulted in unethical outcomes. It has become more difficult to conduct clinical research because of economic reasons. The rules for research seem to have adjusted to the interests of the billion-dollar pharmaceutical industry. To patent, research, develop, and get approval for a new drug, and then market it, you need a hundred million dollars. Economics may have become more important for universities than conducting good research that benefits people with health problems. A lot of research money is reserved for currently popular, conventional research ideas. Over the past decades it has become increasingly more difficult to get grants for outside-the-box research that could be groundbreaking.[35]

Most medical journals are more or less dependent on industry. Pharmaceutical companies execute strong power over what is published in main medical journals.[36] Design, and thus also results, of clinical trials are affected by industry funding.[37] The power of money is also strong in nutrition research. Dr Lenard Lesser at Children's Hospital in Boston studied funding of research on soft drinks, juice, and milk. He found that industry-funded research was published seven times more often with positive conclusions in comparison with papers lacking industry funding.[38]

The construction of current psychiatric diagnoses has been affected by the power of money. This is shown for anxiety syndromes as a whole,[39] social phobia,[40] and depressive disorder.[41] Many of the participants in The Diagnostic and Statistical Manual of Mental Disorders, Fourth Edition (DSM-IV) task force had substantial economic funding from pharmaceutical industry.[42]

In our culture the belief in medical science actually shares many

PHARMACEUTICAL ADVERTISING BIASES JOURNALS AGAINST VITAMIN SUPPLEMENTS

Orthomolecular Medicine News Service,
February 5, 2009

"[I]n major medical journals, more pharmaceutical advertising is associated with publishing fewer articles about dietary supplements," according to researchers from Wake Forest University School of Medicine and the University of Florida. In fact, more pharmaceutical company advertising resulted in the journal having a greater number of articles with "negative conclusions about dietary supplement safety."

Medical journals with the most drug advertisements "published significantly fewer major articles about dietary supplements per issue than journals with the fewest pharmads (P [less than] 0.01). Journals with the most pharmads published no clinical trials or cohort studies about supplements. The percentage of major articles concluding that supplements were unsafe was 4 percent in journals with fewest and 67 percent among those with the most pharmads (P = 0.02)." The authors concluded that "the impact of advertising on publications" is real, and said that "the ultimate impact of this bias on professional guidelines, health care, and health policy is a matter of great public concern."

Positive reports about the effects of high-dose vitamins have long been ignored by the medical establishment instead of being further examined scientifically.

1. Kemper, K. J., K. L. Hood. "Does Pharmaceutical Advertising Affect Journal Publication about Dietary Supplements?" *BMC Complement Altern Med.* 8(11) (Apr 9, 2008). Full text at http://www.biomedcentral.com/1472–6882/8/11 or http://www.pubmedcentral.nih.gov/articlerender.fcgi?tool=pubmed&pubmedid=18400092.

similarities with religion. This was described by David F. Horrobin in his book *Science is God* in the following way: "Science is the modern god. . . . the position of science in the mid-twentieth-century parallels that of religion in the mid-nineteenth. . . . Twentieth-century scientists, like nineteenth-century theologians, make the wildest claims on behalf of their god, not realizing the danger that if these claims are proved false their god may fall."[43]

Olivier Clerc also argued that the medical establishment as a modern-time religion is allied with the government powers, as the Catholic Church once was.[44]

As pointed out by Hugh D. Riordan: "Only within its full historical, social, political, cultural, and economic context can anything be fully understood . . ."[45] It is important to look at the whole picture. That modern medicine is a new religion and bad science has become big business may be sad, but we need to face this reality and use our own brains to make sound decisions for our health.

Evidence-Based Medicine (EBM)

Although the term was not used in a scientific paper until 1992,[46] the concept of evidence-based medicine began much earlier. Its main principles have been described as follows: (1) scientific documentation, (2) clinical practice, (3) patient values and wishes, and (4) other relevant circumstances.[47]

This description could be compatible with good science. However, EBM is often described in media and general debate as only the first of these characteristics. In this way EBM has obtained a more restricted meaning, limited in scientific respect and deviating from good clinical practice. This departure from the original principles of EBM would be better called eminence-based medicine.[48] Chapter 4 describes the current state of evidence-based medicine in detail.

EVIDENCE-BASED MEDICINE: NEITHER GOOD EVIDENCE NOR GOOD MEDICINE

by Steve Hickey, Ph.D. and Hilary Roberts, Ph.D.

Evidence-based medicine (EBM) is the practice of treating individual patients based on the outcomes of huge medical trials. It is, currently, the self-proclaimed gold standard for medical decision-making, and yet it is increasingly unpopular with clinicians. Their reservations reflect an intuitive understanding that something is wrong with its methodology. They are right to think this, for EBM breaks the laws of so many disciplines that it should not even be considered scientific. Indeed, from the viewpoint of a rational patient, the whole edifice is crumbling.

The assumption that EBM is good science is unsound from the start. Decision science and cybernetics (the science of communication and control) highlight the disturbing consequences. *EBM fosters marginally effective treatments, based on population averages rather than individual need.* Its mega-trials are incapable of finding the causes of disease, even for the most diligent medical researchers, yet they swallow up research funds. Worse, EBM cannot avoid exposing patients to health risks. It is time for medical practitioners to discard EBM's tarnished gold standard, reclaim their clinical autonomy, and provide individualized treatments to patients.

The key element in a truly scientific medicine would be a rational patient. This means that those who set a course of treatment would base their decision-making on the expected risks and benefits of treatment to the individual concerned. If you are sick, you want a treatment that will work for you, personally. Given the relevant information, a rational patient will choose the treatment that will be most beneficial. Of course, the patient is not in isolation but works with a competent physician, who is there to help the patient. The rational decision making unit then becomes the doctor-patient collaboration.

The idea of a rational doctor-patient collaboration is powerful. Its main consideration is the benefit of the individual patient. However, EBM statistics are not good at helping individual patients—rather, they relate to groups and populations.

The Practice of Medicine

Nobody likes statistics. Okay, that might be putting it a bit strongly but, with obvious exceptions (statisticians and mathematical types), many people do not feel comfortable with statistical data. So, if you feel inclined to skip this article in favor of something more agreeable— please wait a minute. For although we are going to talk about statistics, our ultimate aim is to make medicine simpler to understand and more helpful to each individual patient.

The current approach to medicine is "evidence-based." This sounds obvious but, in practice, it means *relying on a few large-scale studies and statistical techniques* to choose the treatment for each patient. Practitioners of EBM incorrectly call this process using the "best evidence." In order to restore the authority for decision-making to individual doctors and patients, we need to challenge this orthodoxy, which is no easy task. Remember Linus Pauling: despite being a scientific genius, he was condemned just for suggesting that vitamin C could be a valuable therapeutic agent.

Historically, physicians, surgeons and scientists with the courage to go against prevailing ideas have produced medical breakthroughs. Examples include William Harvey's theory of blood circulation (1628), which paved the way for modern techniques such as cardiopulmonary bypass machines; James Lind's discovery that limes prevent scurvy (1747); John Snow's work on transmission of cholera (1849); and Alexander Fleming's discovery of penicillin (1928). Not one of these innovators used EBM. Rather, they followed the scientific method, using small, repeatable experiments to test their ideas. Sadly, practitioners of modern EBM have abandoned the traditional experimental method, in favor of large group statistics.

What Use are Population Statistics?

Over the last twenty years, medical researchers have conducted ever larger trials. It is common to find experiments with thousands of subjects, spread over multiple research centers. The investigators presumably believe their trials are effective in furthering medical research. Unfortunately, despite the cost and effort that go into them, they do not help patients. According to fundamental principles from decision science and cybernetics, large-scale clinical trials can hardly fail to be wasteful, to delay medical progress, and to be inapplicable to individual patients.

Much medical research relies on early twentieth-century statistical methods, developed before the advent of computers. In such studies, statistics are used to determine the probability that two groups of patients differ from each other. If a treatment group has taken a drug and a control group has not, researchers typically ask whether any benefit was caused by the drug or occurred by chance. The way they answer this question is to calculate the "statistical significance." This process results in a p-value: the lower the p-value, the less likely the result was due to chance. Thus, a p-value of 0.05 means a chance result might occur about one time in twenty. Sometimes a value of less than one-in-one-hundred (p [less than] 0.01), or even less than one-in-a-thousand (p [less than] 0.001) is reported. These two p-values are referred to as "highly significant" or "very highly significant" respectively.

Significant Does Not Mean Important

We need to make something clear: in the context of statistics, the term *significant* does not mean the same as in everyday language. Some people assume that "significant" results must be "important" or "relevant." This is wrong: the level of significance reflects only the degree to which the groups are considered to be separate. Crucially, the significance level depends not only on the difference between the studied groups, but also on their size. So, as we increase the size of the groups, the results become more significant—even though the effect may be tiny and unimportant.

Consider two populations of people, with very slightly different average blood pressures. If we take ten people from each, we will find no significant difference between the two groups because a small group varies by chance. If we take a hundred people from each population, we get a low level of significance (p [less than] 0.05), but if we take a thousand, we now find a very highly significant result. Crucially, the magnitude of the small difference in blood pressure remains the same in each case. In this case a difference can be *highly significant* (statistically), yet in practical terms it is extremely small and thus effectively insignificant. In a large trial, highly significant effects are often clinically irrelevant. More importantly and contrary to popular belief, the results from large studies are less important for a rational patient than those from smaller ones.

Large trials are powerful methods for detecting small differences. Furthermore, once researchers have conducted a pilot study, they can perform a power calculation, to make sure they include enough subjects to get a high level of significance. Thus, over the last few decades, researchers have studied ever bigger groups, resulting in studies a hundred times larger than those of only a few decades ago. This implies that the effects they are seeking are minute, as larger effects (capable of offering real benefits to actual patients) could more easily be found with the smaller, old-style studies.

Now, tiny differences—even if they are "very highly significant"—are nothing to boast about, so EBM researchers need to make their findings sound more impressive. They do this by using *relative* rather than *absolute* values. Suppose a drug halves your risk of developing cancer (a relative value). Although this sounds great, the reported 50 percent reduction may lessen your risk by just one in ten thousand: from two in ten thousand (2/10,000) to one in ten thousand (1/10,000) (absolute values). Such a small benefit is typically irrelevant, but when expressed as a relative value, it sounds important. (By analogy, buying two lottery tickets doubles your chance of winning compared to buying one; but either way, your chances are miniscule.)

The Ecological Fallacy

There is a further problem with the dangerous assertion implicit in EBM that large-scale studies are the best evidence for decisions concerning individual patients. This claim is an example of the ecological fallacy, which wrongly uses group statistics to make predictions about individuals. There is no way [a]round this; even in the ideal practice of medicine, EBM should not be applied to individual patients. In other words, EBM is of little direct clinical use. Moreover, as a rule, the larger the group studied, the less useful will be the results. A rational patient would ignore the results of most EBM trials because they aren't applicable.

To explain this, suppose we measured the foot size of every person in New York and calculated the mean value (total foot size/number of people). Using this information, the government proposes to give everyone a pair of average-sized shoes. Clearly, this would be unwise—the shoes would be either too big or too small for most people. Individual responses to medical treatments vary by at least as much as their shoe sizes, yet despite this, EBM relies upon aggregated data. This is technically wrong; *group statistics cannot predict an individual's response to treatment.*

EBM Selects Evidence

Another problem with EBM's approach of trying to use only the "best evidence" is that it cuts down the amount of information available to doctors and patients making important treatment decisions. The evidence allowed in EBM consists of *selected* large-scale trials and meta-analyses that attempt to make a conclusion more significant by aggregating results from wildly different groups. This constitutes a tiny percentage of the total evidence. Meta-analysis rejects the vast majority of data available, because it does not meet the strict criteria for EBM. This conflicts with yet another scientific principle, that of not selecting your data. Rather humorously in this context, science students who select the best data, to draw a graph of their results, for example, will be penalized and told not to do it again.

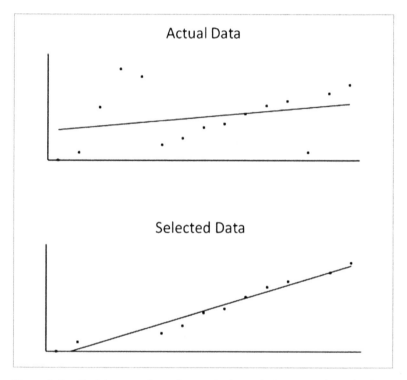

One of the first lessons for science students is to not select the best evidence; all data must be considered. The lines indicate how using just the "best" data gives a better, though misleading, fit.

More EBM Problems

The problems with EBM continue. It breaks other fundamental laws, this time from the field of cybernetics, which is the study of systems control and communication. The human body is a biological system and, when something goes wrong, a medical practitioner attempts to control it. To take an example, if a person has a high temperature, the doctor could suggest a cold compress; this might work if the person was hot through over-exertion or too many clothes. Alternatively, the doctor may recommend an antipyretic, such as aspirin. However, if the patient has an infection and a raging fever, physical cooling or symptomatic treatment might not work, as it would not quell the infection.

In the above case, a doctor who overlooked the possibility of infection has not applied the appropriate information to treat the condition. This illustrates a cybernetic concept known as *requisite variety*, first proposed by an English psychiatrist, Dr. W. Ross Ashby. In modern language, *Ashby's law of requisite variety* means that the solution to a problem (such as a medical diagnosis) has to contain the same amount of relevant information (variety) as the problem itself. Thus, the solution to a complex problem will require more information than the solution to a straightforward problem. Ashby's idea was so powerful that it became known as the *first law of cybernetics*. Ashby used the word *variety* to refer to information or, as an EBM practitioner might say, evidence.

As we have mentioned, EBM restricts variety to what it considers the "best evidence." However, if doctors were to apply the same statistically-based treatment to all patients with a particular condition, they would break the laws of both cybernetics and statistics. Consequently, in many cases, the treatment would be expected to fail, as the doctors would not have enough information to make an accurate prediction. Population statistics do not capture the information needed to provide a well-fitting pair of shoes, let alone to treat a complex and particular patient. As the ancient philosopher Epicurus explained, *you need to consider all the data.*

Restricting our information to the "best evidence" would be a mistake, but it is equally wrong to go to the other extreme and throw all the information we have at a problem. Just as Goldilocks in the fairy-tale wanted her porridge "neither too hot, nor too cold, but just right" doctors must select just the right information to diagnose and treat an illness. The problem of too much information is described by the quaintly-named *curse of dimensionality*, discussed further below.

A doctor who arrives at a correct diagnosis and treatment in an efficient manner is called, in cybernetic terms, a *good regulator*. According to Roger Conant and Ross Ashby, every good regulator of a system must be a model of that system. Good regulators achieve their goal in the simplest way possible. In order to achieve this, the diagnostic processes must model the systems of the body, which is why doctors undergo years of training in all aspects of medical science. In addition, each patient must be treated as an individual. EBM's group statistics are irrelevant, since large-scale clinical trials do not model an individual patient and his or her condition, they model a population—albeit somewhat crudely. They are thus not good regulators. Once again, a rational patient would reject EBM as a poor method for finding an effective treatment for an illness.

Real Science Means Verification

As we have implied, science is a process of induction and uses experiments to test ideas. From a scientific perspective, therefore, we trust but verify the findings of other researchers. The gold standard in science is called Solomonoff Induction, named after Ray Solomonoff, a cybernetic researcher. *The power of a scientific result is that you can easily repeat the experiment and check it.* If it can't be repeated, for whatever reason (because it is untestable, too difficult, or wrong), a scientific result is weak and unreliable. Unfortunately, EBM's emphasis on large studies makes replication difficult, expensive, and time consuming. We should be suspicious of large studies, because they are all but impossible to repeat and are therefore unreliable. EBM asks us to trust its results but, to all intents and purposes, it precludes replication. After all, how many doctors have $40 million dollars and five years available to repeat a large clinical trial? Thus, EBM avoids refutation, which is a critical part of the scientific method.

In their models and explanations, scientists aim for simplicity. By contrast, EBM generates large numbers of risk factors and multivariate explanations, which makes choosing treatments difficult. For example, if doctors believe a disease is caused by salt, cholesterol, junk food, lack of exercise, genetic factors, and so on, the treatment plan will be complex. This multifactorial approach is also invalid, as it leads to the curse of dimensionality. Surprisingly, the more risk factors you use, the less chance you have of getting a solution. This finding comes directly from the field of pattern recognition, where overly complex solutions are consistently found to fail. Too many risk factors mean that noise and error in the model will overwhelm the genuine information, leading to false predictions or diagnoses. Once again, a rational patient would reject EBM, because it is inherently unscientific and impractical.

Medicine for People, Not Statisticians

Diagnosing medical conditions is challenging, because we are each biochemically individual. As explained by an originator of this concept, nutritional pioneer Dr. Roger Williams, *"Nutrition is for real people. Statistical humans are of little interest."* Doctors must encompass enough knowledge and therapeutic variety to match the biological diversity within their population of patients. The process of classifying a particular person's symptoms requires a different kind of statistics (Bayesian), as well as pattern recognition. These have the ability to deal with individual uniqueness.

The basic approach of medicine must be to treat patients as unique individuals, with distinct problems. This extends to biochemistry and genetics. An effective and scientific form of medicine would apply pattern recognition, rather than regular statistics. It would thus meet the requirements of being a good regulator; in other words, it would be an effective approach to the prevention and treatment of disease. It would also avoid traps, such as the ecological fallacy.

Personalized, ecological, and nutritional (orthomolecular) medicines are converging on a truly scientific approach. We are entering a new understanding of medical science, according to which the holistic approach is directly supported by systems science. Orthomolecular medicine, far from being marginalized as "alternative," may soon become recognized as the ultimate rational medical methodology. That is more than can be said for EBM.

(Used with permission of the authors. Orthomolecular Medicine News Service, December 7, 2011. Available online at: http://orthomolecular.org/resources/omns/v07n15.shtml)

ABOUT THE AUTHORS

Steve Hickey holds a Ph.D. in Medical Biophysics from the University of Manchester, England. He has carried out research in the fields of medical imaging, biophysics, pattern recognition, artificial intelligence, and decision science. Hilary Roberts has her Ph.D. in the effects of early-life undernutrition from the Department of Child Health at the University of Manchester, England. She also holds degrees in computer science, physiology, and psychology.

For Further Reading

Hickey, S., H. Roberts. *Tarnished Gold: The Sickness of Evidence Based Medicine.* CreateSpace, 2011.

Orthomolecular Medicine News Service. "Pharmaceutical Advertising Biases Journals Against Vitamin Supplements." Orthomolecular.org. February 5, 2009. http://orthomolecular.org/resources/omns/v05n02.shtml. (accessed July 2012)

Orthomolecular Medicine News Service. "Free, Peer-Reviewed Nutritional Medicine Information Online: No Evidence, Eh?" Orthomolecular.org. October 3, 2011 http://orthomolecular.org/resources/omns/v07n08.shtml. (accessed July 2012)

SUMMARY

"Believe those who are seeking the truth.
Doubt those who find it."
—ANDRÈ GIDE, (1869–1951);
NOBEL PRIZE IN LITERATURE 1947

The use of the expression evidence-based medicine without defining its meaning is common. This leads to confusion and manipulation to such an extent that the concept EBM has been compromised. A detailed critique finds the EBM approach "diametrically opposite in both theory and practice to the real scientific gold standard."[1]

In the development of medical drugs a hierarchy of study designs for evaluation of intended effects of therapy is often presented in this order:

1. Randomized controlled trials

2. Prospective follow-up studies

3. Retrospective follow-up studies

4. Case-control studies

5. Anecdotal: case report and series

As pointed out by Jan P. Vandenbroucke, professor of clinical epidemiology at Leiden University, The Netherlands, the hierarchy is reversed in study designs for discovery and explanation:

1. Anecdotal: case reports and series, findings in data, literature

2. Case-control studies

3. Retrospective follow-up studies

4. Prospective follow-up studies

5. Randomized controlled trials

As the author points out, we need both the hierarchy of discovery and explanation as well as the hierarchy of evaluation.[2]

CHAPTER 5

ORTHOMOLECULAR MEDICINE AND BIOCHEMICAL INDIVIDUALITY

*"Let thy food be thy medicine,
and thy medicine be thy food."*
—HIPPOCRATES (460–370 B.C.)

Emphasizing the importance of food as a basic element in prevention and treatment of disease, orthomolecular medicine (OM) is a tradition with ancient roots. Specifically, OM is about using molecules known to the human body for thousands of generations. The word orthomolecular was introduced by Linus Pauling[1] and became known after his paper in *Science* (1968).[2] It means "correct molecule," and refers to the practice of using optimal amounts of the nutrients and substances naturally found in foods or produced by our bodies for disease prevention and treatment.

NUTRITIONAL BIOCHEMISTRY

Why are nutrients of interest in treatment and prevention of disease? It is easy to understand why these essential substances are necessary when it comes to the classic deficiency diseases. For other illnesses, however, the primary prescriptions used in current medical treatment are for patented medications, most of which are xenobiotic molecules. These substances are not orthomolecular, but are foreign to our bodies in some way. In the treatment of a disease in a specific patient, medical drugs may be better or worse than a more natural, orthomolecular approach. Patented pharmaceutical drugs have been most successful for acute (short-term) medical states such as infections, most clearly seen since the introduction of antibiotics in the 1940s. But nutrition, physical exercise, and stress management are important parts of an integrated treatment plan for the treatment of chronic, long-term disease.

Why do medical drugs such as antidepressants affect the body? They interact with receptors in our nervous system. Receptor systems have developed over many million years. These and other biochemical structures have evolved in continuous interplay with the nutrients received into the body and the endogenous substances synthesized in the body, in our complicated biology. Thus, our receptors are shaped for nutrient-built substances and not for pharmaceutically created drugs. Because of this, medical drugs are often modified copies of orthomolecular substances.

Our individual, specific types of receptors may vary in quantity and sensitivity, however, depending on our genetics and environmental factors. Receptors and other biochemical systems in the body are also continually affected by outer and inner environmental factors such as body temperature, pH, food, toxins, radiation, disease, social, psychological and physical stress, light, physical activity, and cultural aspects.

Nutrients build our bodies and provide its structure and function. Our genes interact with the environment and using our nutritional intake support the synthesis of proteins, lipids, hormones, neurotransmitters, enzymes, and other substances within the body. Serotonin and norepinephrine (noradrenalin) have been considered the most important neurotransmitters in causing (and preventing) depression. These molecules are built in our bodies from amino acid precursors, in cooperation with some vitamins and minerals. L-tryptophan is converted to 5-HTP and then into serotonin. L-tyrosin converts to L-dopa, then into dopamine, and then into norepinephrine. We also need several cofactors for these biochemical reactions to take place: the vitamins B_3, B_6, folic acid, B_{12}, C, and D, and the minerals magnesium, zinc, iron, and copper. All of these substances, and other essential nutrients, are required for healthy production of these neurotransmitters and for our mental health. They can be provided in the diet as well as in supplements. A healthy diet may be enough for many people to prevent depression, but knowledgeable supplementation is most helpful if you want to use nutrition for depression treatment.

Nutrients can have many effects on our biochemistry. In different amounts and combinations they can produce exciting health benefits, as demonstrated by the history of orthomolecular medicine, which today is contributing to evidence-based nutrition (EBN).[3]

BIOCHEMICAL INDIVIDUALITY

When in doubt, use nutrition first.
—ROGER WILLIAMS (1893–1988)

We are all different. Not only that we look different, we walk and talk differently. Our genes are different. But, how about one-egg (identical) twins? Their DNA is quite similar, but not totally identical.[4]

The expression *chemical individuality* (in German) was used by professor Carl H. Huppert, who emphasized the chemical differences between species in a rectorial address delivered on November 15, 1895 at the Carl Ferdinand University in Prague.[5] This address was later credited by Archibald Garrod (1857–1936), who published a paper "Chemical Individuality" in *The Lancet* in 1902.[6] Later he became better known for coining the term "inborn errors of metabolism." In the same way that William Osler is remembered for revolutionizing modern methods of diagnostics, Archibald Garrod had an enormous importance for the study of the underlying mechanisms of disease. But the person who really introduced the concept of *biochemical individuality* was Roger J. Williams (1893–1988). His book *Biochemical Individuality* was first published in 1956.[7]

In recent years new terms with comparable meanings have been used. One of these is *genomic individuality.*[8] Another, more common, expression is *personalized medicine.* Biochemical individuality is a core concept in orthomolecular medicine. To this we may also add the concept of *nutritional individuality.*[9] Indeed, the differences in each of us range from the obvious (visible and behavioral) to the ultramicroscopic (chemical and nutritional). These differences are very important. Combining this understanding with the knowledge that there are also different mechanisms for each individual in the development, course, and healing of depression will give us a foundation for sound evaluation and treatment.

With this fully in mind, we turn to the part of the book you have been waiting for: what can we *do* about it all? How can we use the orthomolecular approach to treat depression?

PART TWO

ACTION

CHAPTER 6

AN EVOLUTION-BASED HEALTH PROGRAM

*"Patients should have rest, food, fresh air,
and exercise—the quadrangle of health."*
—WILLIAM OSLER (1849–1919)

Ever since Hippocrates, many have promoted and implemented lifestyle programs for initial treatment of disease or health problems. This is also useful in depression. It must not replace conventional evaluation and treatment if the depressive state is serious, dangerous, long-standing, or otherwise complicated, but it can be a valuable adjunct even in these cases. There are eight basic elements in our version of this approach. Depression and other chronic diseases are multifactorial, so it is usually beneficial to consider combined treatment measures that incorporate some or all of the following:

1. **Knowledge.** This is the foundation for personal responsibility and attitude, and is necessary if you want real change. It consists of general knowledge from the life sciences, but it also includes specific knowledge about you, your illness and symptoms, your history, limits, resources, dreams, and hopes. No one else—doctors, nutritionists, experts, or government bodies—can give you all this. Do your own research! You need knowledge to make informed decisions related to your health. With knowledge you can take responsibility. You may consult and get some knowledge from experts, but never trust them blindly.

2. **Nutrition.** Healthy food is natural food without added sugar, artificial sweeteners, taste, color, and other substances added for improved consistency or as preservatives. It means regular and balanced eating. Good nutrition is also important for a natural gut bacterial flora, from which we get several B vitamins. Food supplements like vitamins, minerals, trace elements, fatty acids, amino acids, enzymes, and probiotics also support an optimal nutritional intake.

3. **Light.** Historically speaking, being indoors most of the day is a new behavior for humans. Daytime sunshine is essential, as is darkness (lights out!) at nighttime.

4. **Sleep and daily rhythm (often referred to as circadian or diurnal rhythm).** A natural rhythm with light/darkness and wakefulness/ sleep is basic for health and well-being. Sleep is necessary for physiological recovery. One hundred years ago electricity was a luxury and it was easy to have a natural daily rhythm. Our modern 24-7 society makes this basic need surprisingly difficult.

5. **Exercise.** Physical activity, moving, and getting outdoors is important. Behavioral activity counteracts depression. Choose the type of activity you like—enjoyment is important for persistence.

6. **Stress management.** Learning and practicing stress reduction, acceptance, and commitment help you navigate when under stress. Some people benefit from meditation or yoga. Spending some time in nature is a good stress reliever.

7. **Emotional connections.** Good relationships with other people (or pets), love, and friendship have all been proven to enhance health and improve quality of life.

8. **Community involvement.** Outside work and social and cultural interests and commitment can improve mood and outlook.

The table below describes these aspects:

TWENTY-FIRST-

	STONE AGE	CENTURY LIFE	HEALTH PROGRAM
Knowledge	Directly applied for survival and primary needs	Complicated, difficult to evaluate in the information society, unevenly distributed	Take responsibility, critically consult different sources of expertise for informed judgment and decision
Nutrition	Unrefined nutrient-dense species-adapted food from nature	Added sugar and artificially refined food, with man-made contaminants	Use natural food and optimal supplements according to biochemical individuality
Light	Outdoor life	Indoor life	Take optimal time outdoors and in sunshine
Sleep	Rhythm adjusted to the celestial bodies; sleep patterns adapted to natural periods of light and dark	Electric light available at all times of day, disrupting natural rhythms	Keep a regular sleep schedule for physiologic recovery
Exercise	High level of physical activity	Less physical activity due to use of motor vehicles and work tools	Maintain a regular moderate exercise program, possibly outdoors, to stimulate endorphins and other biochemical systems
Stress	Natural emotional response to acute stress situations	Continuous (chronic) high-stress level leading to persistent tension and hormone imbalances	Practice stress management techniques for stress reduction, including acceptance, commitment, hope, optimism, and realism
Emotional Relations	Family-related in traditional societies	Fragmented relationships in an anonymous global society	Keep healthy emotional relationships within circles of family and friends
Community Involvement	Natural engagements within traditional society	Scattered commitments in a demanding, hierarchical community	Maintain a satisfactory working life, social and cultural involvement

This table describes our evolution-based treatment for health problems. The program works in harmony with conventional treatment of disease. It can and should be integrated with other kinds of treatments when they are indicated. The application of this health plan must be individualized for each person's particular situation.

We cannot go back to Stone Age living, but to a very large extent we still have Stone Age genes. The mismatch between our genes and twenty-first century life is the main explanation for the changed illness scenario we have today. The health plan above supports our inherent healing mechanisms. Its eight aspects relate to our evolutionary-based needs, physiology, and biochemistry, and aims to balance hormones and activate the nervous system. This seems common sense, but it is an often omitted perspective in "modern" health care.

Similar programs are being described more and more frequently. A similar program for people with depression was described by Robert J. Hedaya, professor at Georgetown University.[1] He promotes a balanced nutrition plan, an exercise program, and spiritual renewal as the essential aspects to enhance the benefits and beat the side effects of conventional medication. Similar holistic approaches were proposed by David Servan-Schreiber, formerly clinical professor of psychiatry at the University of Pittsburgh School of Medicine,[2] and Stephen Ilardi, associate professor in clinical psychology at Duke University, Lawrence, Kansas.[3] Another self-help book was written by Harvard Medical School psychiatrists Arthur Barsky and Emily Deans.[4] All of these programs can help people take responsibility for their health through lifestyle changes, even if the nutritional aspects of the programs are less developed.

INDIVIDUALIZED HEALTH PLAN

Use the following chart to analyze your individual needs when developing your own personal health plan. The fourth column can be used for evaluation after an optional number of weeks or months.

YOUR LIFE TODAY DATE:	DESIRED OR PLANNED CHANGES	SELF-RATED EVALUATION, DATE

Knowledge	What do you know about your health?	What more would you like to learn about your health?
Nutrition	How and what do you eat? What do you not eat and why? Supplements?	Would you like to change how/what you eat?
Light	How long do you get outdoors, daily?	Is this something you would like to change?
Sleep	How much and when do you sleep?	Would you like to change your sleep pattern?
Exercise	How physically active are you?	Would you like to change your exercise pattern?
Stress management	Is your life stressful?	Would you like to change your reaction to stress?
Emotional relations	Do you have close emotional relationships?	Would you like to change your relationships to others?
Community/ societal involvement	Do you have any societal commitment?	Would you like to change your work, social, or cultural commitments?

Diverse Depression Destroyers

The following suggestions have four things in common: They have nothing to do with vitamins; they are cheap; they often work, and they cannot hurt to try!

- **Sit under a pine tree.** This is said to have worked for Native Americans; it might work for you. Maybe it is the pine tree. Maybe it is sitting on Mother Earth. Maybe it is just the sitting. I (AWS) was raised steeped in American Indian lore since I was six. You can thank the Rochester, New York YMCA's Camp Hiawatha for it. Back in 1961, our summer Y camp groups were organized, by age, into historically accurate named tribes. Six-year-olds like me were usually Navahos. The older kids were in several individual Iroquois nations. We met together for "councils" in front of hand-carved totem poles. We heard Indian stories around the campfire. We learned Indian dances and Indian songs, and received feathers for sporting achievements. (I also had the camp record for eating the most blueberry pancakes, but I digress.) As the years have passed, I have grown to increasingly appreciate "primitive" ideas like this one. So try a tree, or better yet, immerse yourself in a whole group of them.

- **Get some sunshine.** I live in upstate New York, between Rochester and Buffalo, two of the cloudiest locales in America, so I appreciate the value of getting enough sunshine. It may take more conscious effort depending upon your location, but it is a proven mood booster wherever you live.

- **Carbohydrates relieve depression.** Sugar will make you feel better . . . for a very short time, and we are talking minutes. Then you will feel much worse for several hours. Do not eat sugar—no matter what your problem, sugar will make it worse. Complex whole-grain carbohydrates, on the other hand, will make you feel better for a good while, and without a sugar rebound.

- **Exercise relieves depression.** This is well established in the medical literature, but rarely implemented by depressed people. It's understandable if you are too sick and tired to move, but get off your keester and do it anyway. Do isometrics or yoga. Put on an exercise video, turn the sound way up, and just do it. Lift weights. Get outdoors. Walk. Run. Paddle. Pedal. Chop wood. Walk to the grocery store and walk home with your groceries.

- **Do some charitable work.** Try altruism. Serve humankind. As Bullwinkle, reciting a poem, so aptly advised, "Do something for somebody, quick!" Helping others lifts depression elegantly. Volunteer at a soup kitchen or homeless shelter. Pitch in at your local food bank. A new perspective on life is guaranteed.

Nearly thirty years ago I was volunteering a small bit of time at

St. Joseph's House of Hospitality in inner-city Rochester, New York. Even then, St. Joe's, as it is locally known, fed about a hundred poor people daily. Not everyone who comes in for the free lunch is starving, but some are. At the beginning of the first sitting, I happened to see one little boy, about six years old or so, who really seemed to be looking forward to his meal that day. I saw what he had set in front of him: an enormous helping of a simple type of goulash (macaroni, hamburger, tomato sauce). "Are you really going to eat all that?" I asked him, smiling. "Yes I am," he answered, with a far bigger smile. And he was right, too. Did that kid ever eat. He finished his first heaping plateful so fast he must have inhaled it. He had seconds, and thirds, and quite possibly fourths that I wasn't fast enough to see. I had never witnessed a child eat that much before, and my own kids had hefty appetites of their own, let me tell you. The impression this made on me was pretty strong.

- **Lift your Spirit.** Get more involved with your local church. Don't have a church, or synagogue, mosque, or temple? Visit a few. When I was a lonely college student, far from home in a whole new place, I went, by myself, into a conveniently located church on Sunday morning. Before I left, I had offers for dinner at several parishioners' homes and I was in the church choir. That truly lifted my spirits. In my opinion, it is the kindness of the people that makes the faith real.

- **Do stuff you enjoy.** Walk away from stuff you do not enjoy. Easier said than done, we know. But one young woman was greatly benefited by simple advice from her therapist: If things get too tough, just say "Can't deal," and walk away. A lot of bar fights have been avoided that way.

- **Visit your local animal shelter.** Adopt a dog. Get a kitten. Get a rabbit. No, not in the same lap. But try petting an animal. Many institutions have an official, resident dog on the staff. I (AWS) saw a nursing home dog actually making the rounds. He was a beautiful, gentle Golden Retriever. He knew what he was doing, too. He'd stop at each bed, at each chair, for about a minute. He'd let the resident pet him, and then he'd move on and check the next patient. Yes, as an ethology (animal behavior biology) student, I was thoroughly taught that we should not anthropomorphize; that is, do not assume human motives for animal actions. But as a parent, I have had too many pets that would literally check on my children at bedtime to deny that animals are brighter than we sometimes tell each other in textbooks. When my daughter's baby cries, her cat has special behaviors depending on the urgency of the cry. Intelligent, compassionate pet stories abound. The take-home lesson? Take home an unwanted pet from your local animal shelter, or claim an unwanted puppy or kitten. (And please be sure to have it neutered.)

- **Count your blessings instead of your SSRI (antidepressant) tablets.** I have been depressed. Who hasn't? The only real variables are cause, frequency, and degree. It has been frequently and rightly said, "We are all in this together." I can almost always find ten things to be thankful for. Once, when my life was a real mess (lost marriage; lost father; lost job), I was only able to come up with five. That was at the very lowest moment of my life. The only good things about having only five blessings to count are that (1) it saves counting time and (2) it beats having only four.

- **Caffeine works, sometimes.** A cup of coffee or tea will give you a lift, and that is a physiological fact. But there are downsides to caffeine consumption. One is that too much is bad for your heart and mind, and very bad for some persons especially sensitive to caffeine. Large maintained intake (more than eight or nine cups of coffee daily) can lead to permanent changes in heart rhythm. Robust caffeine intake has been reported to cause actual put-them-in-a-mental-hospital psychosis.[5] "Too much" is a variable quantity, depending on who you are and where you are physically. As drugs go, caffeine is comparatively safe and, at low levels, only moderately physically addictive.

And try these, too:

- Put yourself in the path of wandering miracles.

- Call friends on the telephone. Share and ask. Go and visit. Community healing works.

- Put on some nice music.

- Turn on one of those horrible television talk shows. Watch and listen to the people and realize how less messed up you are than they are.

- Detoxify. Clean the liver and colon, and you'll be surprised how much peppier you feel. The easiest way to do this is with lots of vegetable juicing.

- Add your idea here: If it works, do it!

CHAPTER 7

FOOD REALLY DOES MATTER

*"If people let the government decide what foods they
eat and what medicines they take, their bodies will soon
be in as sorry a state as are the souls of those
who live under tyranny."*
—THOMAS JEFFERSON (1743–1826), AUTHOR OF
THE *DECLARATION OF INDEPENDENCE*

Once upon a time we were hunter-gatherers. Not long ago foods were homemade and more natural. Food production was small scale, while today it is an industry. If you go hunter-gathering in a big food store you find industry products. Most of these products contain fructose and other sugars, different sweeteners, other tastes, artificial color, and consistency substances—added intentionally. This is nothing less than contamination. These foods are full of empty calories. It means you get enough (or too many) calories for the day, but less of the nutrients you would get from natural foods. Thus, we have gone from malnutrition to dysnutrition.[1]

FOOD RESPONSIBILITY

The interests of food industry, governments, and experts are intertwined, and the results are very present in what is available to us in our modern grocery stores. However, what we decide to eat is critical to the gene-nutrition interaction that occurs in our bodies. Understanding this interface cannot be avoided if you seriously want to find out about health and disease. The bottom line is: what you eat is not something you should leave to big business or to big government. If you are interested in specific solutions for your own, your family's, or your patient's health, you also have to look outside the box, not only inside.

	PSYCHIATRY "INSIDE THE BOX": CONVENTIONAL THERAPY, SUPPORTED BY AUTHORITIES	PSYCHIATRY "OUTSIDE THE BOX": UNCONVENTIONAL (SELF-MANAGED) THERAPY, QUESTIONED BY AUTHORITIES
Biochemical therapy	Patented xenobiotic medical drugs	Orthomolecular substances in food and supplements
Electromagnetic therapy	ECT (electroconvulsive therapy)	Light therapy, negative ions, earthing (including walking barefoot outdoors)
Psychosocial therapy	Psychotherapy	Nature, culture, societal involvement, stress management, exercise, sleep regulation

For best treatment, use both what is inside and outside the box! Obviously, you will have to form your own view on what and how to eat. But, knowledge will give you well-informed choices. Remember, you are not a victim! If health matters to you, so will food. It has long been accepted that food is an important factor in obesity, diabetes, coronary heart disease, and many other diseases. However, it is commonly said that the food you eat is not important in depression. The psychiatric profession has had a strong resistance toward recognizing a "food/mental health" relationship, although it seems self-evident to a lot of people. Depression is a biochemical process, and food affects human biochemistry. Every molecule in our body is built from what we eat, drink, and breathe. Food matters, and our bodies are built from food matter.

What's Best?

*"The composition of each meal could have a direct effect
on the production of chemical signals in the brain."*
—THE NEW YORK TIMES, JANUARY 9, 1979

The value of different kinds of foods is often heatedly debated. There is no one food that is best for everyone. We are biochemically different. For example, there are several genes related to obesity. One of these, the fat mass and obesity-associated gene (FTO), is associated with obesity and influences appetite regulation. In one study those having this gene were more susceptible to obesity if they combined a high-fat diet with low physical activity.[2] Other researchers showed that obese women with normal insulin sensitivity lost weight easier with a high-carbohydrate and low-fat diet, but those with decreased insulin sensitivity lost weight easier on a low-carbohydrate and high-fat diet.[3]

Especially since the 1980s, government authorities have recommended that people consume a major proportion of their calories from carbohydrates. For some people this may be no problem at all. However, for a lot of people with diabetes or other expressions of the metabolic syndrome, the reverse is true: decreasing their carbohydrate intake is beneficial. People with depression or other disorders of the nervous system need optimal amounts of healthy fats and protein.

Lots of people consume fast foods. This means empty calories and a high carbohydrate intake. The estimated per capita sugar consumption in different countries correlates with their prevalence rates of depression.[4] In a cross-sectional population-based survey of 5,498 tenth-grade students in Oslo, Norway, high consumption

> Remember: No supplement, indeed, no therapy of any kind, will work unless you stop eating sugar and start eating whole, unprocessed, natural foods.

levels of sugar-containing soft drinks were associated with mental distress, conduct problems, and hyperactivity.[5] Decreased insulin resistance has been linked to increased suicide rates[6] and depression.[7]

In recent years respected psychiatric journals have published scientific papers pointing to significant relationships between food and mood. A prospective Spanish study suggested that a Mediterranean dietary pattern had a preventive effect for depressive disorders.[8] In the Whitehall II prospective cohort (demographic study) of over ten thousand working men and women, a "processed food" diet (heavily loaded with sweetened desserts, fried food, processed meat, refined grains, and high-fat dairy products) was a risk factor for middle-age depression in comparison to a "whole food" diet (heavily loaded with vegetables, fruits, and fish).[9] Two Australian papers are also noteworthy. In an epidemiological study of women, a "traditional" dietary pattern characterized by vegetables, fruit, meat, fish, and whole grains was associated with a lower risk for depression or anxiety disorder. However, a "Western" diet of processed or fried foods, refined grains, sugary products, and beer was associated with more psychological symptoms.[10] The author commented that "reverse causality and confounding cannot be ruled out as explanations." In a later investigation of adolescents, a healthy diet at the beginning of the study was related to better mental health. Changes in diet during the study predicted later psychological functioning. Thus, "results did not support the reverse causality hypothesis."[11]

THYROID

Physicians of depressed patients need to be sure to rule out thyroid insufficiency. Don't let yourself be a thyroid android; that is, a robot-like, near-catatonic personality simply because of thyroid insufficiency.

I (AWS) have all too personally seen what thyroid, or a lack of it, can do. My mother suffered from arthritis, depression, skin problems, fatigue, unexplained weight gain, and assorted other miserable symptoms in her early fifties. Nothing seemed to help until she got a new family physician. He promptly put her on thyroid medication, and she was a new woman. Her singing voice came back, along with her get-up-and-go. Her weight came down, her joy of living came up, and her skin looked great. No more bags under the eyes; no more three-hour daily naps. If this is you, then perhaps a thyroid supplement (by prescription) is for you.

The Thyroid Stimulating Hormone (TSH)
Test Is Inadequate

"For thirty years I was a zombie with every low thyroid symptom, but a "normal" TSH, so I was told my thyroid was not the problem. Finally my body started shutting down (I started to feel dead), hair falling out and blood pressure sky-high. I borrowed some dessicated natural thyroid and started treating myself. Immediately I began to recover but the HMO refused to give me a prescription. They even wrote me a letter telling me to discontinue it! The mental and physical suffering were so great, also realizing I had lost so many years. Eventually I got a prescription for desiccated natural thyroid. I had to save my own life."

The biggest mistake a doctor can make is to disbelieve a patient. This goes triple for thyroid symptoms.

Desiccated/Extract versus Synthetic Thyroid

If you are one of the millions who struggle with depression, you may also be one of the millions who suffer from subtle low-thyroid conditions. Some physicians literally laugh patients out of the office when they ask about thyroid supplementation. But thyroid supplementation can be a reasoned, compassionate, alternative to just "learning to live with it."

There is an important difference between T_3 and T_4 thyroid hormone. T_3 (triiodothyronine) seems to be the one to watch. Doctors characteristically over-emphasize your T_4 (l-thyroxine, or "storage" thyroxine) level and effectively ignore T_3 (fast-acting or "active" thyroxine) levels. Physician fixation on test results' numbers, which are inadequate to detect borderline conditions, results in masses of people suffering with the symptoms of low thyroid. These all-too-common symptoms include fatigue, depression, weight gain, insomnia, difficult menopause, endometriosis, and quite a variety of other symptoms, including arthritis and rheumatic complaints, low sex drive, infertility, and skin problems.

What to do? First of all, if you are depressed, or just feel crummy in general, insist on thyroid testing and get a copy of your test results. By law, your doctor must provide test results to you if you ask. So ask!

Interpretation of the tests is the key. Since a "normal" or even somewhat high T_4 can coexist with the symptoms of low thyroid function, do not accept a test for T_4 alone. Insist on T_3 testing as well, and pay special attention to it. TSH testing will almost always be done when thyroid testing is performed. High TSH levels means that the brain and pituitary (gland) are asking for more thyroid hormone. Some orthomolecular physicians consider any TSH number over 3.0 to be suspicious, and anything over 4.0 merits treatment if symptoms are present.

DOCTORS AND SYNTHETIC THYROID

Carol L. Roberts, M.D., writes:

"The synthetic form of thyroid replacement, Synthroid, is a form of T_4, a "prohormone" that must be converted by the body to the active form, T_3. Many people have a hard time making this conversion, due to genetic abnormalities, nutritional deficiencies, or missing enzymes in their system . . . . [Natural thyroid] is made from desiccated [dried] pig thyroids, and contains both T_4 and T_3 as well as other components of the whole gland . . . more natural, more effective option. Most doctors won't prescribe it because Synthroid is what they learned about in medical school and they are not about to move beyond their training. For the few who do, they use dosages that are about half what the patient needs . . . ."

From: "The FDA Does Away with Armour Thyroid: Another Example of Freedom of Choice in Healthcare Being Taken Away" *Creative Loafing, Tampa* September 2, 2009 http://cltampa.com/dailyloaf/archives/2009/09/02/the-fda-does-away-with-armour-thyroid-another-example-of-freedom-of-choice-in-healthcare-being-taken-away#.TzZS_eQncik (accessed July 2012)

With tests done, be prepared to require your doctor to take action. Request a therapeutic trial of thyroid supplement. If you do not need it, you will promptly show symptoms of too much thyroid. These include rapid heartbeat, unusual difficulty sleeping, sweating and otherwise feeling hot, hyperactivity, a racing mind, nervousness, and twitching. If you have these symptoms, lower the dose, or halt the trial. If you feel better, then you needed the supplement.

NATURAL THYROID INFORMATION

The product description for Armour Thyroid indicates that thyroid hormone should be used with caution in patients with angina pectoris or the elderly because they have a greater likelihood of occult cardiac disease. (http://www.armourthyroid.com) Cardiovascular symptoms will require a decrease in dosage. Thyroid hormone may complicate diabetes and its treatment, the use of oral anticoagulants, and should be used with caution with young children.

Additional biochemical details may be found at: http://www.frx.com/pi/Armourthyroid_pi.pdf

Some other brands of natural desiccated thyroid, sometimes known as thyroid extract are:

- Thyroid from Erfa Canada (http://thyroid.erfa.net/)

- NP Thyroid from Acella Pharmaceuticals (http://npthyroid.com)

- Nature-Throid (http://npthyroid.com), and

- Westhroid (http://npthyroid.com) are from RLC Labs (http://rlclabs.com)

- A list including other brands can be found at: http://www.stopthethyroidmadness.com/armour-vs-other-brands/

Note: the authors have no financial connection whatsoever with the manufacturers of any thyroid product or food supplement.

Recommended Reading

Shames, R. L., K. H. Shames. *Thyroid Power: Ten Steps to Total Health*. New York: HarperCollins, 2001.

YOUR OWN NATURAL NEUROTRANSMITTERS

Those of us who have experienced the depths of clinical depression know just how awful it really is. When you are in the bag, it is hard to think out of the bag. But there is a way out.

One all-too-fashionable way is through the use of drugs called Selective Serotonin Uptake Inhibitors (SSRI). Prozac is the most famous, but there are a number of them, including:

- Citalopram (Celexa)
- Escitalopram (Lexapro)
- Fluoxetine (Prozac, Prozac Weekly, Sarafem)
- Paroxetine (Paxil, Paxil CR, Pexeva)
- Sertraline (Zoloft)
- Fluoxetine combined with the atypical antipsychotic olanzapine (Symbyax)

The sneaky thing about SSRI treatment is that it often works very well . . . for a while. Long-term SSRI use is not safe and ultimately is unlikely to be successful. Rather than give a synthetic drug to enhance, block, or mimic the body's chemical nerve messengers (neurotransmitters), it is possible to encourage the body to make them naturally, using nutrition.

If we are what we eat, then our nerves also depend on what they are fed. Eating the right foods offers tremendous potential for the alleviation of depression and related disorders.

Make Your Own Norepinephrine

A depletion of the neurotransmitter called norepinephrine may result in poor memory, loss of alertness, and clinical depression. The chain of chemical events in the body that creates this substance is:

L-phenylalanine (from protein foods) → L-tyrosine (made in the liver) → dopa → dopamine → norepinephrine → epinephrine

This process looks complex but actually is easily accomplished, particularly if the body obtains plenty of vitamin C. The dietary supply of the first ingredient, L-phenylalanine, is usually adequate, so it is more likely to be a shortage of vitamin C that limits one's production of norepinephrine. Physicians who have given large doses of vitamin C to their patients have had striking success in reversing depression. It is a remarkably safe and inexpensive approach to try.

In a double-blind case study tyrosine supplementation had a clear antidepressant effect.[12]

Make Your Own Acetylcholine

Acetylcholine is the final neurotransmitter of your parasympathetic nerve system. This means that, among other things, it facilitates good digestion, deeper breathing, and a slower heart rate. You may perceive its effect as "relaxation."

Your body makes its own acetylcholine from choline. Choline is available in the diet as phosphatidyl choline, which is found in lecithin. Lecithin is found in egg yolks and most soy products. Three table-spoons daily of soya lecithin granules provide about five grams (5,000 milligrams) of phosphatidyl choline. Long-term use of this amount is favorably mentioned in *The Lancet*.[13] Lecithin supplementation has no known harmful effects whatsoever. In fact, your brain, by dry weight, is almost one-third lecithin. How far can we go with this idea of simply feeding the brain what it is made up of? In *Geriatrics,* July 1979, leci-thin is considered as a therapy to combat memory loss. Studies at the Massachusetts Institute of Technology show increases in both choline and acetylcholine in the brains of animals after just one lecithin meal. According to an article in *Today's Living,* supplemental choline has even shown promise in treating Alzheimer's disease.[14]

Lecithin is good for you. How good? Each tablespoon (7.5 grams) of lecithin granules contains about 1,700 milligrams (mg) of phospha-tidyl choline, 1,000 mg of phosphatidyl inositol, and about 2,200 mg of essential fatty acids in the form of linoleic acid. It also contains the valuable omega-3 alpha linolenic acid, which is a precursor to the lon-ger fatty acid molecules found in fish oil. It is the rule, not the excep-tion, that one or more of these valuable substances is undersupplied in our daily diet.

Lecithin tastes crummy. How crummy? Well, the lecithin that is available in capsules is the most popular form of supplementary lec-ithin. These are sold at health food stores and are admittedly conve-nient, but they are also expensive. And—you would have to take eight to twelve capsules to get the value of even one tablespoon of lecithin!

Since a normal supplemental dose is three or more tablespoons daily, that's a lot of capsules to swallow. Much less costly is liquid lecithin. A taste for liquid lecithin has to be acquired, shall we say. It is easier to take if you first coat the spoon with milk or molasses. After taking liquid lecithin, it is wise to have a "chaser" of any dairy product or, again, molasses.

Probably the best way to get a lot of lecithin easily is to take lecithin *granules*. Stir the granules quickly into juice or milk. They won't dissolve but rather will drift about as you drink. Lecithin granules can also be used as a topping on any cold food—ice cream comes to mind. Also, they are not bad if stirred into yogurt. If you put lecithin granules on hot food they will melt, and you will then have liquid lecithin.

Beef and sheep brains are also an excellent source of lecithin, but don't expect us to recommend them. All the supplemental forms of lecithin above are made from soybeans. An alternate non-soy source is egg yolk. Generally, maximum benefit is obtained when you eat the yolk lightly cooked (such as in a soft-boiled egg).

By the way, the correct pronunciation of *lecithin* is "less-a-thin." This is easy to remember because you probably are less-a-thin than you used-to-a-be.

Make Your Own Serotonin

Tryptophan is made into serotonin, one of your body's most potent neurotransmitters. Serotonin is responsible for feelings of well-being and mellowness. Serotonin has such a profound effect that Prozac, Paxil, and similar antidepressants artificially keep the body's own serotonin levels high. You can do the same thing naturally through diet by eating high-tryptophan foods, a list of which follows later in this chapter. And no one can tell us that beans, peas, cheese, nuts, sunflower seeds, and good ol' wheat germ are toxic if you eat a lot of them.

Plenty of carbohydrates in your meals helps tryptophan get to where it does the most good: your brain, because they are required in order to cross the blood-brain barrier. So cheese and crackers provide a better effect than the cheese standing alone. Cover your ears, animal friends, for I am also about to condone eating the occasional dead bird. Poultry, especially the dark meat, is a rich (yet very cheap) source of tryptophan. Add potatoes or stuffing, and you have the reason everybody is sprawled out and snoring up a storm after a typical Thanksgiving food orgy. But to be able to look your parakeet in the eye after the fourth Thursday in November, you can stay vegetarian and still get tanked up on tryptophan.

Five servings of beans, a few portions of cheese or peanut butter, or several handfuls of cashews provide 1,000–2,000 mg of tryptophan. This will work as well as prescription antidepressants—but don't tell the drug companies. Some skeptics think that the pharmaceutical people already know, and that is why the FDA is less than enthusiastic about tryptophan supplements. Here are two quotes in evidence:

> Pay careful attention to what is happening with dietary supplements in the legislative arena. . . . If these efforts are successful, there could be created a class of products to compete with approved drugs. The establishment of a separate regulatory category for supplements could undercut exclusivity rights enjoyed by the holders of approved drug applications.
>
> —FDA Deputy Commissioner for Policy David Adams,
> at the Drug Information Association Annual Meeting, July 12, 1993

> The task force considered many issues in its deliberations including to ensure that the existence of dietary supplements on the market does not act as a disincentive for drug development.
>
> —FDA Dietary Task Force Report, released June 15, 1993

Tryptophan is one of the ten essential amino acids you need to stay alive. It is added to liquid feedings for the elderly and all infant formulas by law. This says a great deal about its safety, as well as its importance.

And, tryptophan is really quite easy to get from the good foods listed below.

So go, eat, and be happy!

FOODS HIGH IN THE AMINO ACID
L-TRYPTOPHAN

The numbers below refer to milligrams of L-tryptophan per 100-gram (3.5 ounce) portion, which is about the size of a deck of playing cards. This is not a large serving; you might easily double or triple the amounts listed below in a single meal. Note that vegetarian sources are as good as, and often much better than, flesh sources.

Beans

Dried peas	250	Pinto beans	210
Lentils	215	Red kidney beans	215
Navy beans	200	Soy beans	525

Nuts and Seeds

Brazil nuts	185	Pumpkin seeds	560
Cashews	470	Sesame seeds	330
Filberts	210	Tahini	
Peanuts	340	(ground sesame seeds)	575
Peanut butter		Sunflower seeds	340
(natural, not commercial)	330		

Other nuts generally provide at least 130 mg per small serving, usually more.

Grains

Wheat germ	265

Cheese

Cheddar	340	Parmesan	490
Swiss	375		

Other cheeses tend to be lower in tryptophan but are still very good sources.

Eggs	210
Poultry	250
Brewer's Yeast	700

(Source: USDA, Amino Acid Content of Foods)

Meats are generally regarded as a good source of tryptophan, organ meats supposedly containing the highest amounts. However, most meats are in the range of 160–260 mg per 100 grams, with organ meats ranging between 220 and 330 mg. These figures certainly do not compel meat eating. They do compel split pea, cheese, and cashew eating!

If you want to use a supplement to increase serotonin you may wish to chose 5-HTP (5-hydroxytryptophan). This molecule is a metabolic intermediate between the essential amino acid L-tryptophan and the neurotransmitter serotonin. As a support for synthesis of serotonin it is good to supplement with the cofactors vitamin B_6 (50–200 mg), vitamin C (several thousand mg in divided doses), magnesium (500 mg) and zinc (30–50 mg). These daily doses are approximate. Your own levels should be determined with the cooperation of your physician.

CHAPTER 8

ORTHOMOLECULAR TREATMENT

"It's supposed to be a secret, but I'll tell you anyway.
We doctors do nothing.
We only help and encourage the doctor within."
—ALBERT SCHWEITZER, M.D., (1875–1965),
NOBEL LAUREATE

As drugs and psychotherapy may be of limited value for an individual person, it is important to develop other methods of treatment, preferably oriented toward the causes of depression and its consequences. Orthomolecular treatment uses macronutrients in the form of natural food and micronutrients in suitable combinations, tailored to a specific individual. The research referred to in this chapter is often based on studying single nutrients, as this has been the mainstream research tradition. However, orthomolecular medicine usually combines complex nutrient formulas. This is further discussed later in this book.

DISCOVERY AND PROGRESS IN VITAMIN RESEARCH

The biochemist Casimir Funk (1884–1967) coined the term vitamin (vital amine) to describe compounds vital to health. Historically, the group of vitamins we find commonly described today were successively discovered (1897–1941), isolated (1928–1948), structurally elucidated (1930–1956), and synthesized (1894–1972).[1] To this point the ruling concept was "vitamins as prevention."

Vitamins as Prevention

This view was based on the belief that vitamins are needed in only small amounts as catalysts, which are recycled in the body almost indefinitely. Vitamins are needed only for prevention of deficiency diseases. However, this idea was later replaced with a new concept as further discoveries were made.

ONE READER WRITES:

My dear husband suffered with chronic "clinical depression" for nine years. He's had every standard psychotropic—each one having its own nice little package of side effects. In Australia, one particular newish drug is recommended as having "few side effects"—my husband's GP [general practitioner] gives him a free sample to try, kindly left in his office by the drug rep. An eight page document about this drug is offered to patients, *only on request.* Go to the United States website of the manufacturer, and you may download a fifty-seven page document listing the *known* pre- and post-marketing side effects, one of which is "death." We were already on the road to better nutrition (love those mung beans!) when we came across the *FoodMatters* movie and your mention of niacin for treating depression. Niacin? The vitamin B complex? Really? Could it be so simple? I have done a lot of research in the last year. I work in a state government mental "health" facility. I am of course just a layperson, but what I know now from the "inside" about psychiatry: talk about quackery! I can access the DSM-IV online in the course of my work. My husband had to undergo assessment by two psychiatrists while he was off work. One hour in their office, and a questionnaire later, and apparently he suffers from a number of psychological disorders that have somehow escaped my attention during our fourteen years of wonderfully close marriage!

   On 3,000 mg [milligrams] of B_3 a day, and within just three days, my husband is completely off his psychotropics, and he's feeling good! I now have back the man I married fourteen years ago. The learning journey we have been on in the last year has been incredible. We really do need to be our own health experts.

Vitamins as Treatment

In 1955 high-dose niacin was shown to decrease increased serum cholesterol.[2] A new paradigm emerged which is called "vitamins as treatment." This idea uses optimum doses of nutrients for both prevention and treatment of diseases. Instead of generic recommended doses applicable to the whole population, it was recognized that the need for a specific vitamin is individualized, based on biochemical differences.

It is important that in higher doses these nutrients have other properties than those previously described as "vitamin functions." New knowledge of the mechanisms of vitamin therapy and treatment options is continuously being developed.

> Modern medicine is primarily a study of what happens when toxic drugs are administered to malnourished bodies.

Vitamins as Competition

It has been said that pharmaceutical medicine has little to gain from a cheap vitamin cure that cannot be patented and exploited for high profit. Observers have also witnessed what happens to medical doctors who have defected to drugless healing: they gain many grateful patients but lose a lot of research funding. Few pharmaceutical companies willingly contribute to their competition.

Vitamin Dosages

Effective doses are high doses, often 1,000 times more than the United States Recommended Dietary Allowance (RDA) or Daily Reference Intake (DRI). It is a cornerstone of medical science that dose affects treatment outcome. This premise is accepted with pharmaceutical drug therapy, but not with vitamin therapy. Most unsuccessful vitamin research has used inadequate, low doses. Low doses do not get clinical results.

Investigators using vitamins in high doses have consistently reported excellent results. High doses were advocated almost immediately after individual vitamins were isolated and years before they were commercially available.

A Short History of Vitamin Cures

Heard this one before? "If vitamin therapy was that good, doctors would tell their patients to take a lot of it." It is surprising how many physicians now recommend supplements. What's that? Your doctor still doesn't? Why? Decades of physicians' reports and controlled studies support the use of very large doses of vitamins.

Vitamins have been identified and isolated for about 100 years. While thiamine (B$_1$) is known as the first vitamin discovered, the B vitamin biotin did not have a recommended intake until 1980, more than forty years after it was discovered. The B vitamin folic acid has only been added to processed foods since 1998. There was no RDA whatsoever for vitamin E until 1968.

And now, over four decades after the first men landed on the moon, medical journals and mass media alike would still have you believe that (1) vitamins are not needed in quantity; (2) vitamins are deadly if you exceed government-ordained minimums; and (3) much more research is needed before your doctor should be permitted to use vitamin therapy. As has so often been the case historically, the government and medical industries persist in error today.

What is odd is that decades of physicians' reports and controlled studies support the use of very large doses of supplemental vitamins. The medical literature has ignored nearly seventy-five years of laboratory and clinical studies on high-dose nutrient therapy.

Nutrition therapy pioneer Evan Shute, M.D., wrote of his experiences advocating vitamin E back in the 1940s:

"It was nearly impossible for anyone who valued his future in Academe to espouse a vitamin, prescribe it or advise its use. That would make a man a 'quack' at once. This situation lasted for many years. In the United States, of course, the closure of the J.A.M.A. pages against us and [vitamin treatment] meant that it did not exist. It was either in the U.S. medical bible or it was nought. No amount of documentation could budge medical men from this stance. Literature in the positive was ignored and left unread. Individual doctors often said: 'If it is as good as you say, we would all be using it.'"

FORTY YEARS OF VITAMIN CURES

Notable early medical pioneers of high-dose vitamin research achieved astonishing clinical results quite a long time ago. They published— they were ignored. The following timeline illustrates the discoveries made by these researchers.

1935: Claus Washington Jungeblut, M.D., Professor of Bacteriology at Columbia University, first publishes on vitamin C as prevention and treatment for polio.

—In the same year Jungeblut also shows that vitamin C inactivates diphtheria toxin.

1936: Evan Shute, M.D. and Wilfrid Shute, M.D. demonstrate that vitamin E-rich wheat germ oil cures angina.

1937: Jungeblut demonstrates that ascorbate (vitamin C) inactivates tetanus toxin.

1939: William Kaufman, M.D., Ph.D. successfully treats arthritis with niacinamide (B$_3$).

1940: Drs. Shute publish that vitamin E prevents fibroids and endo-metriosis, and is curative for atherosclerosis.

1942: Ruth Flinn Harrell, Ph.D. measures the positive effect of added thiamine (B$_1$) on learning.

1945: Vitamin E is shown to cure hemorrhages in the skin and mucous membranes, and to decrease the diabetic's need for insulin.

1946: Vitamin E is shown to greatly improve wound healing, includ-ing skin ulcers. It is also demonstrated that vitamin E strengthens and regulates heartbeat, and is effective in cases of claudication, acute nephritis, thrombosis, cirrhosis, and phlebitis.

—William J. McCormick, M.D., shows how vitamin C prevents and also cures kidney stones.

1947: Vitamin E is successfully used as therapy for gangrene, inflammation of blood vessels (Buerger's disease), retinitis, and choroiditis.

—Roger J. Williams, Ph.D. publishes on how vitamins can be used to treat alcoholism.[1]

1948: Frederick R. Klenner, M.D., a board-certified specialist in diseases of the chest, publishes cures of forty-one cases of viral pneumonia using very high doses of vitamin C.

1949: Dr. William Kaufman publishes *The Common Form of Joint Dysfunction* on treating arthritis with niacinamide (Vitamin B_3).

1950: Vitamin E is shown to be effective treatment for lupus erythematosus, varicose veins, and in cases of severe body burns.

1951: Vitamin D treatment is found to be effective against Hodgkin's disease (a cancer of the lymphatic system) and epithelioma.

1954: Abram Hoffer, M.D., Ph.D. and colleagues demonstrate that niacin (B_3) can cure schizophrenia.[2]

—The Shutes' medical textbook, *Alpha Tocopherol in Cardiovascular Disease,* is published.

1955: Niacin is first shown to lower serum cholesterol.[3]

1956: Mayo Clinic researcher William Parsons, M.D., and colleagues confirm Hoffer's use of niacin to lower cholesterol and prevent cardiovascular disease.

—Dr. Harrell demonstrates that supplementation of the pregnant and lactating mothers' diet with vitamins increases the intelligence quotients of their offspring at three and four years of age.

1957: William J. McCormick, M.D., publishes on how vitamin C fights cardiovascular disease.

1960: Dr. Abram Hoffer meets Bill W., cofounder of Alcoholics Anonymous, and uses niacin to eliminate Bill's long-standing chronic depression.

1963: Vitamin D is shown to prevent breast cancer.

1964: Vitamin D is found to be effective against lymph nodal reticulosarcoma, a non-Hodgkin's lymphatic cancer.

1968: Linus Pauling publishes the theoretical basis of high-dose nutrient therapy (orthomolecular medicine) in psychiatry in *Science.*

Linus Pauling defined *orthomolecular medicine* as "the treatment of disease by the provision of the optimum molecular environment, especially the optimum concentrations of substances normally present in the human body."

1969: Robert F. Cathcart III, M.D., uses large doses of vitamin C to treat pneumonia, hepatitis, and, years later, AIDS.

1973: Dr. Klenner publishes his vitamin supplement protocol to arrest and reverse multiple sclerosis.

1975: Hugh D. Riordan, M.D., and colleagues successfully use large doses of intravenous vitamin C against cancer.

All this just up to 1975, and these are merely the highlights. For further information about the most recent forty years, one has only to do a quick search the National Library of Medicine's PubMed/MEDLINE online index. There have been literally thousands of positive nutrition supplement studies since 1975.

References

1. Williams, R. J., "Alcoholics and Metabolism." *Sci Am* (Dec 1948):50–53. Williams, R. J., "The Etiology of Alcoholism: A Working Hypothesis Involving the Interplay of Hereditary and Environmental Factors." *Quart J. Stud Alcohol* 7(4) (Mar 1947):567–87. Williams, R. J., L. J. Berry, E. Beerstecher, Jr., "Biochemical Individuality: Genetotrophic Factors in the Etiology of Alcoholism." *Arch Biochem,* 23(2) (Sep 1949):275–90.

2. Hoffer, A., H. Osmond, J. Smythies. "Schizophrenia: A New Approach. II. Results of a Year's Research." *J Ment Sci* 100(418) (Jan 1954):29–45.

3. Altschul, R., A. Hoffer, J. D. Stephen. "Influence of Nicotinic Acid on Serum Cholesterol in Man." *Arch Biochem Biophys* 54(2) (Feb 1955):558–559.

VITAMINS VERSUS
THE PHARMACEUTICAL INDUSTRY?

The use of high doses of vitamins may be the most unacknowledged successful research in medicine. Not only that: if the media are to be believed, vitamins are downright hazardous, if not deadly.

WELL-PUBLICIZED VITAMIN SCARES FEED THE PHARMACEUTICAL INDUSTRY

Chicken Little was in the medical library one day when a journal fell on her head. She read it, and it scared her so much she trembled all over. Why? Because Chicken Little had read of negative studies on vitamins. She was so afraid that half her feathers fell out.

"Help! Help! Vitamins are killing us! I have to go tell the President!"

So she ran in great fright to tell the President. Along the way she met Henny Penny.

"Where are you going, Chicken Little?" said Henny Penny.

"Oh, help! Vitamins are killing us!" said Chicken Little.

"How do you know?" said Henny Penny.

"I read it with my own eyes," said Chicken Little, "And it was on the news, and part of it fell on my head!"

"Vitamins are killing us? This is terrible, just terrible!" said Henny Penny. "We'd better hurry up."

So they both ran away as fast as they could. Soon they met Ducky Lucky.

"Where are you going, Chicken Little and Henny Penny?"

"Vitamins are killing us! Vitamins are killing us!" said Chicken Little and Henny Penny. "We're going to tell the President!"

"How do you know vitamins are killing people?" said Ducky Lucky.

"I read it with my own eyes," said Chicken Little, "And heard it with my own ears on the news, and part of it fell on my head."

"Oh dear, oh dear!" Ducky Lucky. "We'd better run!"

So they all ran down the road as fast as they could. Soon they met Goosey Loosey walking down the roadside.

"Hello there. Where are you all going in such a hurry?"

"We're running for our lives!" said Chicken Little.

"Vitamins are killing us!" said Henny Penny.

"And we're running to tell the President!" said Ducky Lucky.

"How do you know that vitamins are killing people?" said Goosey Loosey.

"I read it with my own eyes," said Chicken Little, "And heard it with my own ears on the news, and part of it fell on my head!"

"Goodness!" said Goosey Loosey. "Then I'd better run with you."

And they all ran in great fright across a field. Before long they met Turkey Lurkey strutting back and forth.

"Hello there, Chicken Little, Henny Penny, Ducky Lucky, and Goosey Loosey. Where are you all going in such a hurry?"

"Help! Help!" said Chicken Little. "Vitamins are killing us!"

"We're running for our lives!" said Henny Penny.

"And by the way, the sky is falling!" added Ducky Lucky.

"So we're running to tell the President!" said Goosey Loosey.

"How do you know?" asked Turkey Lurkey.

"I read it with my own eyes," said Chicken Little, "And heard it on the news with my own ears, and part of it fell on my head!"

"Oh dear!" said Turkey Lurkey. "I always suspected those damned vitamins were dangerous! I'd better run with you."

So they ran with all their might, until they met Pharma Fred the Fox.

"Well, well, well," said Pharma Fred. "Where are all of you rushing off to on such a fine day?"

"Help! Help!" cried Chicken Little, Henny Penny, Ducky Lucky, Goosey Loosey, and Turkey Lurkey all together. "It's not a fine day at all. Vitamins are killing us, the sky is falling, and we're running to tell the President!"

"But of course vitamins are killing you," said Pharma Fred the Fox. "Now all of you calm down. Here, have a Prozac."

Chicken Little, Henny Penny, Ducky Lucky, Goosey Loosey, and Turkey Lurkey each swallowed a few Prozacs, and some Valium for good measure.

"Well then," said Pharma Fred the Fox. "How did you learn of how dangerous those vitamins really are?"

"I read it with my own eyes," said Chicken Little, "And heard it on the news with my own ears, and part of it fell on my head!"

"I see," said Pharma Fred the Fox. "Well then, follow me, and I'll show you right to the President."

So Pharma Fred the Fox led Chicken Little, Henny Penny, Ducky Lucky, Goosey Loosey, and Turkey Lurkey across a field and through the woods. He led them straight to his den, and they never saw the President.

And Foxy Pharma Fred had most a delicious dinner.

Now look here, everyone: The sky is not falling. Vitamins save lives. We are a nation of sick, undernourished, and overmedicated people. Vitamins are not the problem; they are the solution.

There is not even one death per year from vitamin supplements. However, there are at least 100,000 deaths from pharmaceutical drugs each year in the United States, even when they are taken as prescribed.[3]

All deaths caused by drugs and doctors may total as high as one million deaths per year.[4] Do not be buffaloed and do not be bullied about this: if someone tries to scare you from taking vitamins, *ask to see the scientific papers that they base such a warning on.*

And then, read the actual study very carefully. If you do not, it is easy for someone to tell you what to think.

How to Make People Believe Any Anti-Vitamin Scare

Recent much trumpeted anti-vitamin news is the product of pharmaceutical industry payouts. No, this is not one of "those" conspiracy theories. Here's how it's done:

1. **Cash to the study authors.** Many of the authors of a recent negative vitamin E paper[5] have received substantial income from the

pharmaceutical industry. The names are available in the last page of the paper (page 1,556) in the "Conflict of Interest" section. You will not see them in the brief summary at the *JAMA* website. Money received came from a large number of major pharmaceutical companies, including Merck, Pfizer, Sanofi-Aventis, AstraZeneca, Abbott, GlaxoSmithKline, Janssen, Amgen, Firmagon, and Novartis.

2. **Advertising revenue.** Many popular magazines and almost all major medical journals receive income from the pharmaceutical industry by publishing their advertisements. The only question is, how much? Pick up a copy of one of these publications and count the pharmaceutical ads. The more space sold the more revenue for the publication. If you try to find their advertisement revenue, you'll see that they don't disclose it. So, just count the Pharma ads. Look in all different types of publications: *Reader's Digest,* The *Journal of the American Medical Association (JAMA), Newsweek, Time, AARP Today, The New England Journal of Medicine, Archives of Pediatrics,* even *Prevention* magazine, a "health-oriented" publication. Practically any major periodical.

3. **Rigged trials.** Yes, it is true, and yes, it is provable. In a recent editorial, we explained how trials of new drugs are often rigged.[6] Studies of the health benefits of vitamins and essential nutrients also appear to be rigged. This can be easily done by using low doses to guarantee a negative result, and by biasing the interpretation to show a statistical increase in risk.

4. **Bias in what is published or what is rejected for publication.** The largest and most popular medical journals receive a very large portion of their income from pharmaceutical advertising. Peer-reviewed research indicates that this influences what they print, and even what study authors conclude from their data.[7]

5. **Censorship of what is indexed and available to doctors and the public.** Public tax money pays for censorship in the largest online public medical library on the planet: the United States' National Library of Medicine (MEDLINE/PubMed).[8]

Don't Believe It?

Here's a list of just a few of the published facts about the effectiveness of vitamins in treating disease and improving wellness. How well were these pro-vitamin, anti-drug studies covered in the mass media?

- A Harvard study showed a 27 percent reduction in AIDS deaths among patients given vitamin supplements.[9]

- There have been no deaths from vitamins in twenty-eight years. [10]

- Antibiotics cause 700,000 emergency room visits per year, just in the United States.[11]

- Modern drug-and-cut medicine is at least the third leading cause of death in the United States. Some estimates place medicine as the number-one cause of death.[12]

- Over 1.5 million Americans are injured every year by drug errors in hospitals, doctors' offices, and nursing homes. If in a hospital, a patient can expect at least one medication error every single day.[13]

- More than 100,000 patients die every year, just in the United States, from drugs properly prescribed and taken as directed.[14]

Double Standard

Countless comedians have made fun of the incompetent physician who, when called late at night during a life-threatening disease crisis, says, "take two aspirin and call me in the morning." It's no longer funny. One of the largest pharmaceutical conglomerates in the world ran prime-time national television commercials that declared: "Bayer aspirin may actually help stop you from dying if you take it during a heart attack." The company also promotes such use of its product on the Internet.[15]

Daily Aspirin Use is Linked With Pancreatic Cancer

Here's some information you may have not seen: research has shown that women who take just one aspirin a day, "which millions do to prevent heart attack and stroke as well as to treat headaches—may raise their risk of getting deadly pancreatic cancer. . . . Pancreatic cancer affects only 31,000 Americans a year, but it kills virtually all its victims within three years. The study of 88,000 nurses found that those who took two or more aspirins a week for 20 years or more had a 58 percent higher risk of pancreatic cancer." [16] Women who took two or more aspirin tablets per day had an alarming 86 percent greater risk of pancreatic cancer.

Study author Dr. Eva Schernhammer of Harvard Medical School was quoted as saying: "Apart from smoking, this is one of the few risk factors that have been identified for pancreatic cancer. Initially we expected that aspirin would protect against pancreatic cancer."

How about that.

Now, what if there was one—just one—case of pancreatic cancer caused by a vitamin? What do you think the press would have said about that?

The fact is, vitamins are known to be effective and safe. They are essential nutrients, and when taken at the proper doses over a lifetime, are capable of preventing a wide variety of diseases. Because drug companies can't make big profits developing essential nutrients, they have a vested interest in agitating for the use of drugs and disparaging the use of nutritional supplements.

NOBODY DIES FROM VITAMIN SUPPLEMENTS

There was not even one death caused by a vitamin supplement in 2010, according to the most recent information collected by the U.S. National Poison Data System.

The new 203-page annual report of the American Association of Poison Control Centers (AAPCC), published online, shows zero deaths from multiple vitamins; zero deaths from any of the B vitamins; zero deaths from vitamins A, C, D, or E; and zero deaths from any other vitamin.[1] (Download any Annual Report of the American Association of Poison Control Centers free of charge at http://

www.aapcc.org/annual-reports/. The "Vitamin" category is usually near the very end of the report.)

Additionally, there were no deaths whatsoever from any amino acid or dietary mineral supplement.

Three people died from non-supplement mineral poisoning: two from medical use of sodium and one from non-supplemental iron. On page 131, the AAPCC report specifically indicates that the iron fatality was not from a nutritional supplement.

Fifty-seven poison centers provide coast-to-coast data for the National Poison Data System, "one of the few real-time national surveillance systems in existence, providing a model public health surveillance system for all types of exposures, public health event identification, resilience response and situational awareness tracking."[2]

Well over half of the United States population takes daily nutritional supplements. Even if each of those people took only one single tablet daily, that makes 165,000,000 individual doses per day, for a total of over 60 billion doses annually. Since many people take far more than just one single vitamin or mineral tablet, actual consumption is considerably higher, and the safety of nutritional supplements is all the more remarkable.

If vitamin and mineral supplements are allegedly so "dangerous," as the U. S. Food and Drug Administration and the news media so often claim, then *where are the bodies?*

Over a twenty-eight year period, vitamin supplements have been alleged to have caused the deaths of a total of eleven people in the United States. A new analysis of the Poison Control Center's Annual Report data indicates that there have, in fact, been no deaths whatsoever from vitamins . . . none at all, throughout the entire twenty-eight years that these reports have been available.

> Over 60 billion doses of vitamin and mineral supplements per year in the United States, and not a single fatality. Not one.

The American Association of Poison Control Centers attributes annual deaths to vitamins as follows:

2010: zero	2003: two	1996: zero	1989: zero
2009: zero	2002: one	1995: zero	1988: zero
2008: zero	2001: zero	1994: zero	1987: one
2007: zero	2000: zero	1993: one	1986: zero
2006: one	1999: zero	1992: zero	1985: zero
2005: zero	1998: zero	1991: two	1984: zero
2004: two	1997: zero	1990: one	1983: zero

Even if these figures are taken as correct, and even if they include intentional and accidental misuse, the number of alleged vitamin fatalities is strikingly low, averaging less than one death per year for over two and a half decades. In twenty of those twenty-eight years, AAPCC reports that there was not one single death due to vitamins. Still, the Orthomolecular Medicine News Service Editorial Board was curious: Did eleven people really die from vitamins? And if so, how?

Vitamins Not *The* Cause of Death

In determining cause of death, AAPCC uses a four-point scale called Relative Contribution to Fatality (RCF). A rating of 1 means "Undoubtedly Responsible"; 2 means "Probably Responsible"; 3 means "Contributory"; and 4 means "Probably Not Responsible." In examining poison control data for the year 2006, which lists one vitamin death, it was seen that the vitamin's Relative Contribution to Fatality (RCF) was a 4. Since a score of "4" means "Probably Not Responsible," it quite negates the claim that a person died from a vitamin in 2006.

Vitamins Not *A* Cause of Death

In the other seven years that report one or more of the remaining ten alleged vitamin fatalities, studying the AAPCC reports reveals an absence of any RCF rating for vitamins in any of those years. If there is no Relative Contribution to Fatality at all, then the substance did not contribute to death at all.

Furthermore, in each of those remaining seven years, there is no substantiation provided to demonstrate that any vitamin was a cause of death.

If there is insufficient information about the cause of death to make a clear-cut declaration of cause, then subsequent assertions that vitamins cause deaths are not evidence-based. Although vitamin supplements have often been blamed for causing fatalities, there is no evidence to back up this allegation.

References

1. Bronstein, A. C., D. A. Spyker, L. R. Cantilena, Jr., et al. "2010 Annual Report of the American Association of Poison Control Centers' National Poison Data System (NPDS): 28th Annual Report." Clin Toxicol (Phila) 49(10) (Dec 2011). published online at http://www.aapcc.org/dnn/Portals/0/2010%20NPDS%20Annual%20Report.pdf (accessed July 2012).

The vitamin data mentioned above will be found in Table 22B.

2. Orthomolecular.org. "No Deaths from Vitamins: America's Largest Database Confirms Supplement Safety." Orthomolecular News Service (Dec 28, 2011) http://orthomolecular.org/resources/omns/v07n16.shtml (accessed Aug 2012).

VITAMINS: BENEFITS AND EFFECTS ON DEPRESSION

We will now take a look at those vitamins, minerals, and other nutrients that have the greatest interest in relation to depression.

Vitamin B$_1$

Vitamin B$_1$ or thiamine is crucial for energy production from food and also in mitochondria in cells of the body. Thiamine is also important for the nervous system. It is required for acetylcholine production and it has antioxidant properties.

Lack of thiamine can result in the deficiency disease beriberi. It presents with neurologic symptoms as neuropathy, walking difficulties, confusion, severe lethargy and fatigue, or cardiovascular symptoms as tachycardia, dyspnea, and edema. Depression, loss of appetite, weight loss, poor concentration, irritability, and insomnia can also be expressions of deficiency. The need for thiamine increases with smoking, excessive alcohol consumption, eating junk food, and with age. Supplementing thiamine is also suggested in many diseases of the nervous system, such as chronic fatigue, Alzheimer dementia, and alcoholism.

Ten normal young men were given a thiamine-deficient diet and developed depression and irritability. After thiamine supplementation their symptoms rapidly regressed.[17] In an experimental double-blind study of 80 healthy elderly women it was shown that 10 milligrams daily of thiamine significantly increased appetite, energy intake, body weight and general well-being, and decreased fatigue.[18]

David Benton, professor at the University of Swansea, in a study found low thiamine concentrations to be associated with poor mood scores in females.[19] In a later double-blind study 120 female university students with normal thiamine status were given 50 milligrams thiamine or placebo daily. After two months thiamine had improved their mood, reaction times and energy significantly.[20]

Vitamin B$_2$

Vitamin B$_2$ or riboflavin has a role in cell energy production, is an antioxidant, and has anti-inflammatory properties. Riboflavin interacts with other B vitamins and is also a part of mitochondrial function. The older tricyclic antidepressants may deplete vitamin B$_2$ and this can be a reason to supplement riboflavin.

Riboflavin restriction increased depressive scores in an experimental study of only six men.[21] In an investigation of psychiatric patients, those with affective disorders were low in both riboflavin and vitamin B$_6$.[22]

Increase of blood riboflavin concentrations during supplementation was associated with improvement of some depression symptoms.[23]

Vitamin B$_3$

Vitamin B$_3$ occurs in two forms: nicotinic acid (niacin) and nicotinamide (niacinamide). They are dietary precursors for NAD, NADH, NADP and NADPH, all of which are important coenzymes in energy transduction. Complex I in the mitochondria, the power stations of the cell, is actually NAD. NAD is important in cellular signaling,[24] and has been described as a metabolic oscillator for the regulation of metabolism and aging.[25] Niacinamide protects neurons and other cells.[26] Vitamin B_3 participates in the metabolism of polyunsaturated fats and the signal substances serotonin, dopamine, norepinephrine, and GABA, all considered important in depression and anxiety. As more has become known about the complex metabolism of vitamin B_3 it is possible to comprehend how varying doses of this vitamin may result in many different effects.[27]

The deficiency disease of vitamin B_3 is pellagra. Thousands died from it before Joseph Goldberger (1874–1929) proved its cause was a dietary deficiency in 1926. The well-known symptoms of deficiency are diarrhea, dermatitis, and dementia, but it can also cause depression, anxiety, psychosis, and fatigue.

The Niacin Flush

Niacin has the ability to greatly reduce anxiety and depression. Another feature of niacin is that it dilates blood vessels and creates a sensation of warmth, called a "niacin flush." This is often accompanied with a blushing of the skin. It is this "flush" or sensation of heat that indicates a temporary saturation of niacin.

When you flush, you can literally see and feel that you've taken enough niacin, at least for the moment. The idea is to initially take just enough niacin to have a slight flush. This means a pinkness about the cheeks, ears, neck, forearms, and perhaps elsewhere. A slight niacin flush should end in about ten minutes or so. If you take too much niacin, the flush may be more pronounced and longer lasting. If you flush beet red for half an hour and feel weird, well, you took too much.

A large dose of niacin on an empty stomach is certain to cause profound flushing. "With larger initial doses, the flush is more pronounced and lasts longer," says Dr. Hoffer. "But with each additional dose, the intensity of the flush decreases and in most patients becomes a minor nuisance rather than an irritant. Niacin should always be taken immediately after finishing one's meal."

If you are timid about the flush, probably the best way to accurately control the flushing sensation is to start with very small amounts of niacin and gradually increase until the first flush is noticed. One method is to start with a mere 25 milligrams (mg) three times a day, say with each meal. The next day, try 50 mg at breakfast, 25 mg at lunch, and 25 mg at supper. The following day, you might try 50 mg at breakfast, 50 mg at lunch, and 25 mg at supper. And the next day, 50 mg at each of the three meals. The next day, 75 mg, 50 mg, and 50 mg. Then, 75 mg, 75 mg, and 50 mg, and so on. In this way you have increased at the easy rate of only 25 mg per day. One would continue to increase the dosage by 25 mg per day until the flush occurs.

It is difficult to predict a saturation level for niacin because each person is different. As a general rule, the more you hold without flushing, the more you need. If flushing doesn't happen until a high level, then your body is obviously using the higher amount of the vitamin.

Now that you've had your first flush, what's next? Since a flush indicates saturation of niacin, it is desirable to continue to repeat the flushing, just very slightly, to continue the saturation. This could be done three or more times a day. Niacin can be taken to saturation at bedtime, too, to get to sleep sooner at night. You might be asleep before you even notice the flush.

An important point here is that niacin is a vitamin, not a drug. It is not habit forming. Niacin does not require a prescription because it is that safe. It is a nutrient that everyone needs each day. Different people in different circumstances require different amounts of niacin.

Says Dr. Hoffer: "A person's upper limit is that amount which causes nausea, and, if not reduced, vomiting. The dose should never be allowed to remain at this upper limit. The usual dose range is 1,500 to 6,000 mg daily, divided into three doses, but occasionally some patients may need more. The toxic dose for dogs is about 5,000 mg per 2.2 pounds (1 kilogram) body weight. We do not know the toxic dose for humans since niacin has never killed anyone."

Dr. Hoffer is right. Twenty-eight years of nationwide data from the American Association of Poison Control Center fails to document and confirm any deaths from niacin whatsoever. Zero.

Inevitable physician skepticism and questions about niacin's proven safety and effectiveness are best answered in *Orthomolecular Psychiatry: Treatment of Schizophrenia,* edited by David Hawkins, M.D. and

Linus Pauling, Ph.D,[28] and more recently, by *Niacin: The Real Story* by Abram Hoffer, Andrew W. Saul, and Harold D. Foster.[29]

Persons with a history of heavy alcohol use, liver disorders, diabetes, or pregnancy will especially want to have their physician monitor their use of niacin in quantity. Monitoring long-term use of niacin is a good idea for anyone. It consists of having your doctor check your liver function with a simple blood test.

Plain and simple niacin may be purchased in tablet form at any pharmacy or health food store. Tablets typically are available in 100 mg or 250 mg dosages. The tablets are usually scored down the middle so you can break them in half easily. You can break the halves in half, too, to get the exact amount you want.

If a niacin tablet is taken on an empty stomach, a flush will occur (if it is going to occur at all) within about twenty minutes. If niacin is taken right after a meal, a flush may be delayed. In fact, the flush may occur long enough afterward that you forgot that you took the niacin! Don't let the flush surprise you. Remember that niacin does that, and you can monitor it easily.

If you want a flush right away, you can powder the niacin tablet. This is easily done by crushing it between two spoons. Powdered niacin on an empty stomach can result in a flush within minutes. Sustained release niacin is often advertised as not causing a flush at all. This claim may not be completely true; sometimes the flush is just postponed. It would probably be difficult to determine your saturation level with a sustained- or time-released product. They are also more costly. But the biggest reason to avoid sustained-release niacin is that most reports of side effects stem from use of this form.

There is nothing wrong with niacinamide, by the way. That form of vitamin B$_3$ is frequently found in multiple vitamins and B-complex preparations. Niacinamide does not cause a flush at all. It is usually just as effective in inducing relaxation and calming effects. However, niacinamide does not lower serum cholesterol. This is an important distinction to make when purchasing.

It is a good idea to take all the other B-complex vitamins in a separate supplement in addition to the niacin. The B vitamins, like professional baseball players, work best as a team. Still, the body seems to need proportionally more niacin than the other B vitamins. Even the U.S. Recommended Daily Allowance (RDA) for niacin is much more than for any other B vitamin. Many physicians consider the current RDA for niacin of only 20 mg to be way too low for optimum health. While the government continues to discuss this, it is possible to decide for yourself based on the success of doctors who use niacin for their patients every day.

TO FLUSH OR NOT TO FLUSH?

That is a reader's question:

"My question for you is an attempt to clarify what seems to be a difference of opinion about the niacin flush between you and Dr. Hoffer. He had written[1] that the niacin flush is normal with many people and will diminish or go away as the patient continues to use niacin at his recommended level of 3,000 milligrams per day. You, however, state that the flush is an indication of no niacin deficiency.[2] Who is correct or am I misinterpreting one of you?"

Andrew Saul's response:

This is how I look at it: Generally speaking, people in fairly good health usually choose to increase their doses gradually in order to minimize flushing. If they do increase the dose slowly, what I describe is pretty accurate. For instance, I've been taking niacin for years, in daily but varying doses depending on my stress level or dietary intake. I know by the flush when I've had enough for the moment. It is like turning off the hot water when the tub is full enough for a nice bath. Dr. Hoffer is highly experienced with serious psychiatric cases. Such patients have a niacin dependency, not a mere deficiency. Let's let him speak for himself:

Abram Hoffer, M.D., writes:

We are both correct. Most people flush at the beginning and gradually get adapted to it unless they stop for a few days and then resume it. A few cannot ever get used to it, and they take the no-flush preparations. But the intensity of the flush is very variable. Generally people who need it the most flush the least. That includes arthritics, schizo-phrenics, and elderly people with cardiovascular problems. Some schizophrenics do not flush until they get well and then they do. But the presence of the flush or its intensity cannot be uniquely used to measure the need, as there are too many variables such as food in the stomach, whether the drink with it is hot or cold, the kind of food, other medication. Antipsychotics reduce the intensity of the flush as do aspirin and antihistamines.[3]

References

1. Hoffer, A.. "Vitamin B3: Niacin and Its Amide." DoctorYourself.com. http://www.doctoryourself.com//hoffer_niacin.html (accessed November 2012).

2. Hoffer, A., A. W. Saul, H. D. Foster. Niacin: The Real Story. Laguna Beach, CA: Basic Health, 2012, 50–52.

3. The above Dr. Hoffer quotes are from a private communication, April 7, 2002.

Recommended Reading

Hoffer, A. Vitamin B3 and Schizophrenia: Discovery, Recovery, Controversy. Kingston, ONT: Quarry Press, 1998. Review available at: http://www.doctoryourself.com/review_hoffer_B3.html

Hoffer, A. Dr. Hoffer's ABC of Natural Nutrition for Children: With Learning Disabilities, Behavioral Disorders, and Mental State Dysfunctions. Kingston, ONT: Quarry Press, 1999.

B$_3$ Effects in the Body

Niacin, but not niacinamide, reduces high blood lipids.[30] Niacinamide has anti-inflammatory effects.[31] William Kaufman showed that 2 to 4 grams of niacinamide had positive effects in treatment of osteoarthritis.[32] This was confirmed in a randomized controlled trial (RCT) study,[33] but was not followed up.

During the 1950s Abram Hoffer and Humphrey Osmond showed that vitamin B$_3$ could be effective in early treatment of schizophrenia.[34] Some following studies were negative, but they used a very different methodology. Half a century later, a post-mortem study of brains from people diagnosed with schizophrenia found that their niacin receptors were different than those from normal people.[35] It is an intriguing possibility that this may be one mechanistic explanation for the therapeutic effect of niacin that has been documented in patients with schizophrenia.

Niacinamide has antianxiety effects mediated via GABA receptor neurons.[36] Niacin was found to be effective for benzodiazepine withdrawal in one RCT.[37]

Depression as a symptom of pellagra, which is caused by a deficiency of B_3, was described a century ago.[38]

Nicotinic acid was reported to have antidepressant effects within five days in a study by psychiatrist Annette Washburne.[39] The fifteen patients were treated with between 900 and 2,500 milligrams of niacin daily. In one negative study published three years later in the same journal the patients only received 900 milligrams daily.[40] In a study of two cases depression was described following niacin cessation.[41] Niacin in combination with tryptophan is an antidepressant alternative that may be as good as the old antidepressant imipramine.[42] Possible effective antidepressant mechanisms for niacin and niacinamide are reviewed in another case study.[43] The vasodilatory properties of niacin may have treatment value, and there are many possible biochemical effects for both forms of vitamin B_3.

NADH

NADH is a coenzyme that catalyses more than one thousand biochemical reactions in humans. It is essential for DNA repair, is a very strong antioxidant, and it increases adenosine-5'-triphosphate (ATP) energy in the cell.[44] ATP is used as an energy carrier in living cells.

In an open-label study NADH was used in 205 patients with depression, and 93 percent of the patients exhibited a beneficial clinical effect.[45]

Vitamin B_6

Vitamin B_6 (pyridoxine, pyridoxal, and pyridoxamine) has many functions. Among others, it participates in the metabolism of dopamine, norepinephrine, serotonin, tyramine, tryptamine, taurine, histamine, and GABA.[46] As vitamin B_6 is the cofactor in more than 100 enzyme-catalyzed reactions in humans it is also possible to understand that vitamin B_6 has been shown to have positive effects in many disease states.[47] Long-time high-dose intake of this vitamin has been described to give neurological symptoms. It was claimed that 50 mg/day would be the lowest observable adverse effect level,[48] but this study has been discredited for methodological flaws.[49] Up to 200 mg a day there are no validated reports of toxicity, but sensory neuropathy has been described in rare cases when 500 mg a day are taken for several months.[50]

Dietary intake of vitamin B_6 was inversely associated with depressive symptoms in both girls and boys in a Japanese epidemiologic study.[51]

In a systematic review of vitamin B_6 as treatment for depression some support was found for its use in premenopausal women.[52] An explanation could be that vitamin B_6 is involved in metabolism of carbohydrates and gonadal steroids. However, for other forms of depression treatment with this single vitamin has not been shown to be effective. Still, it is reasonable to use vitamin B_6 in combination with other supplements in depression treatment.

Folic Acid

Folate deficiency may increase risk of depression and weaken the effect of antidepressant treatment. Folic acid, the synthetic form of folate, has been shown to support the antidepressant effect of the antidepressant fluoxetine.[53] One research study claimed that 800 micrograms (mcg) of folic acid and 1 mg of vitamin B_{12} is useful supplementation in management of depression,[54] and another paper suggested 2 grams of folic acid.[55]

L-methylfolate is generated from folate with help from the enzyme MTHFR (methylenetetrahydrofolate reductase), and is the active vitamin used at the cellular level in the body. It is important in regulating serotonin, dopamine, and norepinephrine. It may be that L-methylfolate (Deplin) is more efficient than folate, especially in cases of patients with low MTHFR activity because of a genetic polymorphism (variation).[56]

Vitamin B$_{12}$

Vitamin B$_{12}$ (cobalamin) is chemically the most complex vitamin molecule.[57] It is needed for production of the erythrocytes (the red blood cells), the function of the nervous system, and cell metabolism. Vitamin B$_{12}$ is required for neurotransmitter synthesis.[58] In higher doses cobalamin has intracellular antioxidant effects.[59]

The most known cobalamin deficiency disease is megaloblastic anemia. However, the first deficiency symptoms of this disease may be neuropsychiatric symptoms without simultaneous anemia.[60] Vitamin B$_{12}$ deficiency can present as cognitive decline,[61] depression,[62] and in many other ways.[63]

Vitamin B$_{12}$ is found almost exclusively in animal foods. Vegetarians and especially vegans risk deficiency if this is not considered in their diet. Our ability to absorb vitamin B$_{12}$ gets worse as we age. Cobalamin uptake may also be decreased by several medical drugs. Examples are those used for ulcer and dyspepsia (antacids, histamine$_2$-blockers, and proton-pump inhibitors). It is suggested that xenobiotic drug (made of chemicals not normally found in the body) use has increased cobalamin deficiency in the population.

The concentration of vitamin B$_{12}$ in the blood is often measured by doctors. However, it is not well known, even by medical professionals, that a normal blood value does not exclude a lowered level of cobalamin in the cerebrospinal fluid (CSF). So, if B$_{12}$ does not cross the blood-brain barrier efficiently, the brain may be cobalamin deficient. Such an unbalance in cobalamin values has been described in geriatric patients and in patients with depression.[64] CSF analysis is usually impractical in clinical work, however. Instead, lab tests of increased homocysteine and/or methylmalonic acid may point to cobalamin or folate insufficiency.[65] Some people will need higher doses of cobalamin because of an inborn error of metabolism.[66]

Vitamin B$_{12}$ can be effective for people with depression, anxiety, and fatigue. If antidepressant drug treatment has been ineffective, cobalamin deficiency may be an explanation. An initial higher cobalamin level in blood is associated with better recovery from depression.[67]

Vitamin C

Vitamin C (ascorbate) is most known for its antioxidant effects and prevention of scurvy. Depression and fatigue are symptoms found in scurvy. The original deficiency disease scurvy is considered to be uncommon in the industrial world. However, scurvy or subscurvy is found in people with restricted dietary habits, in conjunction with other diseases, and in hospital patients.[68]

Vitamin C is a vital antioxidant in the brain.[69] It is a cofactor in several enzyme reactions, including catecholamine synthesis. Research suggests that ascorbic acid modulates the function of GABA receptors in the central nervous system.[70] Ascorbate also has a role in mitochondrion metabolism[71] and regulation of gene expression.[72]

Our need for vitamin C varies because of haptoglobin polymorphism.[73] This means that certain groups of people, such as the Inuits, who for a long time have lived in certain parts of the world, need a lower intake of ascorbate to avoid scurvy than other groups of people. Also, a study of glutathione polymorphism supports that we have different needs for vitamin C.[74]

Vitamin C exerts most of its functions within the cell and crosses cell membranes via specific transporters.[75] There is a structural similarity between vitamin C and glucose. This sugar molecule and ascorbate compete for transport into the cell, and therefore hyperglycemia may induce intracellular deficiency of vitamin C and latent scurvy.[76]

Stress, anxiety, and excitement can accelerate the depletion of ascorbate. In a group of healthy subjects 3 grams daily of vitamin C improved mood.[77] In an experiment with five prison volunteers, depletion of ascorbic acid induced higher scores on the Minnesota Multiphasic Personality Inventory (MMPI) test scales for depression, hypochondriasis, and hysteria.[78]

Blood levels of vitamin C have been found to be low in many patient groups, such as chronic psychiatric patients, described to have "subscurvy" characterized by depression and irritability.[79] In this study with diverse psychiatric diagnoses, supplementing with just 1 gram of vitamin C daily had a good effect against depressive symptoms. In a hospital study with patients who had hypovitaminosis C (vitamin C deficiency) 500 mg of vitamin C twice daily for a week significantly increased mood.[80]

Vitamin D

Vitamin D status is dependent on our sun exposure and intake of marine foods. Deficiency is more common for people living far away from the equator. A lack of vitamin D is common, and may contribute to many diseases.[81] This vitamin is also important for brain development and function.[82] Receptors and metabolizing enzymes for vitamin D are present in the central nervous system and other organs. In a study of healthy volunteers, Ubbenhorst found a significant correlation between vitamin D and the personality factors of extraversion and openness.[83]

Some studies support the hypothesis that low levels of vitamin D may increase the risk for depression, but more controlled studies are needed on this topic. A double-blind Australian study found that supplementing healthy subjects with 400 International Units (IU) of vitamin D_3 for five days significantly enhanced mood during winter.[84] In a Baltimore study one single dose of 100,000 IU of vitamin D_2 was significantly more effective than phototherapy for a group of patients with seasonal affective disorder (SAD).[85]

Treatment with vitamin D is suggested especially during the winter season for people living far away from the equator, for people with a lifestyle that provides low skin exposure to the sun, or if low blood levels of vitamin D have been measured.[86] There is insufficient knowledge to say how important vitamin D deficiency is in causing depression, but a limited number of intervention trials support vitamin D supplementation for depression treatment.[87]

Magnesium

This mineral is essential for over 325 enzymatic reactions in the body, many of which are related to production, transport, storage, and use of energy.[88] Magnesium has anti-inflammatory effects. Some of the deficiency symptoms are depression, fatigue, insomnia, stress, anxiety, irritability, anorexia, and muscle cramps. The mean food intake of magnesium has been markedly reduced during the last century. The need for magnesium is higher with physical or mental stress, or if you have a greater intake of calcium (as in milk products) or alcohol.

Magnesium has been described as nature's physiologic calcium blocker.[89] Antidepressant drugs actually inhibit calcium channels.[90] However, calcium channel blockers used as cardiovascular drugs are a possible cause of depression and suicide.[91]

Low levels of magnesium in cerebrospinal fluid (CSF) were found in psychiatric patients who had made suicide attempts.[92] The ratio between magnesium and calcium was decreased in the blood serum and CSF of depressed patients.[93] Serum magnesium levels were significantly lower among depressive compared to control diabetic subjects.[94] Some medical drugs also may lead to hypomagnesemia (low magnesium levels in the blood), probably because of inhibited magnesium absorption. This has been described for proton pump inhibitors.[95] On the other hand, the antidepressants amitriptyline and sertraline increased comparatively low magnesium levels in the erythrocytes (red blood cells) of major depression patients.[96] Increased intracellular magnesium may be part of the mechanism of antidepressants.

An epidemiologic study from Norway found significantly lower depression scores among those consuming more magnesium.[97]

The idea that magnesium has a role in depression treatment is old and rational, but scientific intervention studies are conspicuously few. In 1921 Paul Weston reported at the annual meeting of the American-Medico-Psychological Association (now The American Psychiatric Association) that hypodermic injection of magnesium sulphate was effective in agitated depression.[98] Eby published four successful case studies in which patients with treatment-resistant depression were given 125–300 mg of magnesium with each meal and at bedtime.[99] In the only published randomized treatment trial of this topic, patients with type 2 diabetes, concurrent hypomagnesemia, and depression were randomly allocated and given either the antidepressant imipramine or magnesium chloride solution (equivalent to elemental magnesium 450 mg daily). After twelve weeks both groups had equally recovered significantly.[100] It is reasonable to consider magnesium in depression treatment, especially in treatment-resistant depression.[101]

Zinc

The essential micronutrient zinc is a component of enzymes and other proteins, but is also important as an ionic signal at the cellular level.[102] Many digestive enzymes are zinc-dependent and this is crucial for gastrointestinal uptake of nutrients. Zinc has important regulatory functions in the brain[103] and may increase serotonin uptake in several brain regions.[104] Deficiency may present with skin changes, brittle nails with white spots, slow wound healing, and behavioral disturbances such as hyperactivity, anorexia, and loss of taste. Zinc deficiency is common in the modern diet. The need for zinc increases with a high alcohol intake, but also in strict vegetarians because the high levels of phytic acid in grains and legumes reduce zinc absorption.

Patients with more severe depressions have been reported to have lower serum zinc levels.[105] This has been described as a sensitive marker for treatment-resistant depression.[106] Serum zinc was found to be low in women with postpartum depression.[107]

Depression was found to be related to lower zinc intake and lower serum concentrations of zinc in a study of female students.[108] Another observational investigation suggests that inadequate zinc intake contributes to depressive symptoms in women, and that supplemental zinc is a beneficial adjunct to antidepressants in women.[109] In a third study dietary zinc intake was inverse to depression scores in both male and female Iranian postgraduate students in Malaysia.[110] It is believed that inflammatory processes are important factors in depression, and that zinc deficiency contributes to its cause.[111] In major depression, the incidence of low levels of plasma zinc increased with treatment of the antidepressants amitriptyline and sertraline.[112]

In a double-blind study of young women (age eighteen to twenty-one) 7 mg of zinc and a multivitamin significantly reduced anger and depression scores when compared to a multivitamin alone.[113]

The senses of taste and smell are zinc dependent. A thirteen-year-old girl with anorexia and depression could not smell zinc sulphate. She recovered with its supplementation. This issue recurred when supplementation was discontinued and got better again when zinc was reintroduced.[114] In a double-blind study with anorexic adolescent girls zinc decreased depression symptoms significantly.[115] In another study, patients with major depression had a significantly better response was found compared to placebo when 25 mg of zinc was added to antidepressant medication.[116] With the same dose treatment-resistant depression patients recovered significantly faster when zinc was combined with imipramine compared to imipramine alone.[117] A systematic review of RCTs suggests that zinc is beneficial in depression treatment, either alone or together with antidepressant medication.[118]

Selenium

Selenium is unevenly distributed in the soil, and it is lacking in the local food supply in many parts of the world. Selenium is an ingredient of the enzymes important in the brain, the thyroid, and other organs. The current RDA is 55 mcg. Researchers have suggested that this recommendation should be raised to 75 mcg.[119] As more seleno-enzymes have been discovered it has been argued that a selenium intake as high as 200–300 mcg is needed to maximize the activity of glutathione peroxidase.[120]

In five reviewed studies a low selenium intake was associated with poorer mood.[121] However, in a later treatment study there was no positive effect in people over sixty years of age.[122] In a double-blind RCT 100 mcg of selenium suggested a positive preventive effect against postpartum depression.[123] It has been hypothesized that depression with suicidal behavior in adolescents may be related to alcohol-induced selenium deficiency.[124]

Chromium

Chromium is a trace element required for carbohydrate metabolism. It is part of the glucose tolerance factor (GTF), which also contains niacin and three amino acids. Together with insulin it helps glucose uptake by the cells. Chromium is also important for the brain. In a small study in which older adults received 1,000 mg elemental chromium daily, memory decline was inhibited.[125]

Malcolm McLeod discovered that chromium was therapeutic for one form of depression. One of his patients, George, had long-standing depression and got much better without obvious reason. George told his psychiatrist that he had just started taking a supplement containing different vitamins and minerals. In a single patient double-blind study McLeod found chromium was the effective substance.[126] Early studies suggested that those patients benefitting from chromium also had carbohydrate cravings as a symptom.[127] This is usually found in atypical depression, a less known but nevertheless common form of mood disorder.[128] Atypical features of depression are (1) weight gain or increased appetite; (2) hypersomnia (excessive sleepiness); (3) heavy, leaden feelings in arms or legs; and (4) a long-standing pattern of interpersonal rejection sensitivity resulting in social or occupational impairment.

Two double-blind studies have investigated the use of chromium picolinate for patients with atypical depression who also have carbohydrate craving. In a small study chromium was significantly better.[129] A larger investigation showed no group difference on mood, but appetite and eating increased and carbohydrate craving and diurnal variation of feelings were significantly changed.[130] In the subpopulation with marked carbohydrate craving chromium picolinate showed a significant antidepressant effect.

Omega-3 Fatty Acids

For several decades the health effects of fat have been much debated. When studying the controversy it is clear that opinions in the field often differ from observation and knowledge. Reasons for this can be found in conflicts between cultural tradition, industry, and science. Except for omega-3 fatty acids, there are comparatively few studies on fats and mood. However, all sorts of natural fat—polyunsaturated, monounsaturated, and saturated—together with amino acids and proteins, are necessary for body structure and function. If fear of fats results in avoiding all sorts of fat, it will also decrease the intake of fat-soluble vitamins (A, D, E, and K) and increase associated health risks. The propaganda for lowering cholesterol has been so exaggerated that "fat free" foods and cholesterol lowering drugs have become an enormous uncontrolled experiment. Combined with the increasing refined carbohydrate intake in the modern diet this may have more adverse than healthy effects.[131]

Low cholesterol may actually be a more serious problem than high cholesterol from a psychiatric point of view. Cholesterol is a natural substance abundant in the human nervous system. From cholesterol we synthesize bile acids, steroid hormones, and vitamin D, and it is an essential component of cell membranes. The more cholesterol we consume the less we synthesize in our body, and vice versa. Hypocholesterolemia, low cholesterol in the blood, has been correlated to depression, suicide, impulsivity, and violent behavior. There is some support for a relationship between low cholesterol and serotonin dysfunction in humans.[132] A decreased intake of fats (from 41 to 25 percent of calories) had adverse effects on mood in healthy volunteers.[133] However, there is relatively little research concerning the effects of food on mood.

Polyunsaturated fatty acids are important constituents in the nervous system and in cell membranes in the whole body. We need omega-3 and omega-6 fats in a good balance. George and Mildred Burr showed that a totally fat-free diet resulted in a deficiency disease in rats in 1929.[134] They proved linoleic acid to be an essential dietary component.[135] Later it was established that both linoleic acid (omega-6) and alpha-linolenic acid (omega-3) are essential in humans. These are the building blocks of longer fatty acid molecules required for different functions in normal physiology. The enzymatic transformation from the essential linoleic acid and alpha-linolenic acid is mediated by elongase and desaturase. The efficiency of these chemical reactions depends on several factors, and there is also a variation with genetic polymorphisms of these enzymes. For delta-6 desaturase there is a need for an adequate supply of vitamins B_3, B_6, C, magnesium, and zinc. Cofactors for elongase are vitamins B_3, B_5, B_6, C, and biotin. Conversion into longer-chain polyunsaturated fatty acids is more efficient in fertile women, where sex hormones may be important.[136] Stress hormones have a negative effect on the production and activity of desaturases.[137] Viruses can also inhibit desaturase activity. Polyunsaturated fats are also less stable and more sensitive to oxidative stress compared to saturated fats.

Modern food, together with physical inactivity and stress, is the most important factor for development of metabolic syndrome, which increases the risk of developing cardiovascular disease and type 2 diabetes. For a lot of people today's food contains definitely less omega-3 compared to omega-6 fats. Studies of indigenous people show their intake of omega-3 and omega-6 to be about equal. In industrial countries the intake of omega-3 has decreased, while at the same time the intake of omega-6 has increased so much that people consume between ten and fifty times more omega-6 fats than omega-3 fats. This is important because omega-3 is anti-inflammatory and omega-6 is inflammatory.

Hugh Macdonald Sinclair first proposed that the changing intake of fats may affect diseases of the nervous system in a 1956 paper[138] that many authorities deemed to be much too speculative.[139] Michael Crawford also feared this changed fat intake could be a reason for mental disease.[140] In 1977 David Horrobin suggested that the phospholipid system is important for depression, mania, and schizophrenia.[141] It would take another twenty years before the interest in the relationship between fats and psychiatric disease would become well known. Joseph Hibbeln found a negative correlation between depressions and fish intake in different countries.[142] He also found an inverse relationship between postpartum depression in women and seafood intake during pregnancy.[143]

Basant Puri added ethyl-EPA to the antidepressant treatment of a twenty-one-year-old man who had been depressed for several years. He was much better in a month, and nine months later a magnetic resonance imaging (MRI) scan showed a reduction in the lateral brain ventricular volume.[144] In another case study a thirty-four-year-old pregnant woman with two previous severe depressions refused antidepressant medication. She was given fish oil in a high dose (4 grams of eicosapentaenoic acid (EPA) fish oil and 2 grams of docosahexaenoic acid (DHA) fish oil) and had a good antidepressant effect from it.[145]

Several double-blind RCTs have been conducted to study the antidepressant effect of omega-3 fatty acids. A meta-analysis found fifteen trials from 2002 to 2009 with altogether 916 participants.[146] Supplements containing EPA in quantities greater than or equal to 60 percent of total EPA and DHA showed significant improvement on depression scores, while supplements with EPA with less than 60 percent were ineffective. Effective doses of EPA in excess of DHA (calculated as EPA – DHA) were in the approximate range of 200–2,000 mg per day.

The antidepressant effects of omega-3 fatty acids in a ratio of EPA equal to or greater than 60 percent of total EPA+DHA may be comparatively equal to antidepressant drugs. However, there are other differences. Omega-3 fats have less side effects, more positive healthy side-benefits, are less expensive, and are not environmental toxins.

Side effects from omega-3 fatty acids are uncommon when moderate doses are used. They are also safe to use unless the patient has any bleeding risk.

The positive effects from omega-3 fats may among others be related to their anti-inflammatory mechanisms.[147] Studies show that major depression is often accompanied by immune dysregulation and activation of the inflammatory response system.[148] This may be relevant in depression,[149] other psychiatric disorders,[150] cardiovascular disease,[151] and rheumatoid arthritis.[152]

Thyroid Hormones

In treatment-resistant depression it is not uncommon to use thyroid hormones as augmentation to antidepressant medication. Five of six double-blind studies found triiodothyronine (T_3) to be significantly more effective than placebo in accelerating treatment response.[153] The efficacy of thyroxine (T_4) is less studied and the possible effect comparatively slower.[154] Thyroid hormones were discussed in Chapter 7.

VITAMINS ARE IMPORTANT IN DEPRESSION TREATMENT

Vitamins have a minor role in current mainstream psychiatry. Only when low levels of cobalamin or folate are detected are these specific vitamins commonly prescribed. However, positive results for the treatment and prevention of depression have also been shown with several other nutrients. Nutrients are necessary for building neurotransmitters, enzymes, and everything else in the body. In orthomolecular medicine it is recognized that the natural substances are the most important ones in the long run.

CHAPTER 9

MULTINUTRIENT
TREATMENT

*"If there's a drug that can alter the brain's biochemistry,
there's usually a combination of nutrients that can achieve
the same thing without side effects."*
—CARL C. PFEIFFER (1908–1988)

Historically, it was natural to first study nutrients separately, especially since they were discovered and described at different periods of time. The research model to study each substance individually is also logical. In clinical practice using only one or very few nutrients was sometimes successful. It was the best—and only—treatment if there was a nutrient deficiency. Then, it could also benefit people who needed higher doses of that nutrient, even if they did not have deficiency symptoms.

One example is niacin or vitamin B$_3$. Its deficiency syndrome is pellagra. However, some patients with schizophrenia or anxiety, who have not been diagnosed with vitamin B$_3$ deficiency, will get much better or even cured with niacin in a dose one hundred times the Recommended Daily Intake (RDI). There may be various reasons for this in niacin biochemistry. Possible explanations could be individual differences in absorption in the gastrointestinal tract, transport into the brain, and variations in enzymatic or receptor systems. These aspects are influenced by genetics as well as environment.

However, you will often not see such effective results with just one nutrient. It could be that you do not know which nutrient is needed. A doctor may have laboratory resources that can analyze the levels of some nutrients in the system, but there are others that cannot be determined.

Combinations of vitamins, minerals and other nutrients were used by Max Gerson (1881–1959), who combined vitamins A, B_3, and C, iodine, and potassium for cancer patients.[1] Frederick Klenner (1907–1984) combined vitamins B_1, B_2, B_3, B_6, B_{12}, C, and E, calcium, magnesium, zinc, choline, lecithin, and glycine in his protocol for multiple sclerosis.[2] In the treatment of arthritis William Kaufman (1910–2000) first gave niacinamide, but also combined it with vitamins B_1, B_2, C, and sometimes vitamins A and D.[3]

Several studies have found that a lot of people today may have multiple nutrient deficiencies. U.S. Department of Agriculture studies report that a large percentage of people in the United States do not meet recommended nutrient intake levels. This is related to changes in how we eat and the insufficient nutrient content of food. These combined deficiencies are important factors for a lot of diseases in our world today.

In clinical practice it is obviously a good idea to combine different nutrients instead of just backing one horse. First of all, you won't know what nutrient will help for a specific person before trying. Second, nutrients work together—they cooperate like different players in an orchestra. By now they have been playing in harmony for quite a long time. Some combinations are very natural, considering their role in physiology. Both zinc and magnesium often work together with vitamin B_6, so it is logical to combine them. Third, using single nutrients for an extended period of time may pose a risk for inducing a nutrient imbalance. For example, if you use zinc for a long period, you should consider adding copper. This need is affected by your genetic make-up, the dose and the time it is taken, nutrition, and other life style factors. In a similar way doctors are aware that cobalamin and folate/folic acid are combined, as both participate in methylation, which can be important in depression treatment.[4] A fourth reason for combining a number of nutrients is that it strengthens the antioxidant defense system. In a study of thirty-four healthy subjects, a multinutrient supplement was given for sixteen weeks. By the end of the study their antioxidant vitamin status and enzymatic activities were markedly improved.[5] Bruce

Ames, a well-known Oakland researcher, argued for using a broad range of vitamin and mineral supplements for metabolic tune-up.[6] He later described the *triage theory,* which proposed that modest nutrient deficiencies may increase the risk for diseases of aging.[7]

Vitamin supplementation for one year improved mood for women but not for men in a randomized, double-blind study.[8] The vitamins were: A, B_1, B_2, B_3, B_6, biotin, folic acid, B_{12}, C, and E, at doses ten times what is usually recommended for daily intake. In the study all vitamin concentrations except B_3 were analyzed in the study participants' blood. The findings were that vitamins B_1, B_2, and B_6 were involved in mood improvement. It is of interest that side effects were alike in both the placebo group and the group receiving the supplements, with one exception: nausea was more common in the placebo group. It was concluded that taking these doses of vitamins did not produce adverse effects. An earlier placebo-controlled, randomized controlled trial (RCT) also showed that vitamins B_1, B_2 and B_6 augmented tricyclic antidepressant effect in geriatric depression with cognitive dysfunction.[9]

In another randomized, double-blind, placebo-controlled trial 215 healthy males were given a combination of vitamins and minerals for thirty-three days.[10] Once daily they took a tablet containing 15 mg B_1, 15 mg B_2, 50 mg B_3, 23 mg B_5, 10 mg B_6, 150 mcg biotin, 400 mcg folic acid, 10 mcg B_{12}, and 500 mg C, and 100 mg calcium, 100mg magnesium, and 10 mg zinc. The supplemented group had improved ratings of stress, mental health, vigor, and improved cognitive performance during

HOW SAFE IS VITAMIN C?

If vitamin C were harmful, the entire animal kingdom would be dead. Our nearest primate relatives all eat well in excess of 2,000 milligrams of vitamin C each day. And, pound for pound, most animals actually manufacture from 2,000–10,000 mg of vitamin C daily in their bodies. If such generous quantities of vitamin C were harmful, evolution would have had millions of years to select against it. Vitamin C is not a problem; it is a solution. Linus Pauling personally took 18,000 mg every day.

intense mental processing. The Profile of Mood States (POMS) scores narrowly failed significant change (p=0.054). Similarly, in a double-blind RCT with healthy men between fifty and sixty-nine years of age, a supplement with vitamins (higher than RDI), minerals, and some herbals had a significantly positive effect on a mood, anxiety, and stress scale.[11]

Assuming that inflammation, stress, and mitochondrial function is important in depression it has been suggested that a combination of zinc, N-acetylcysteine, coenzyme Q10, and the omega-3 fatty acid EPA, together with curcumin and resveratrol, should be of interest in depression.[12]

Multinutrient supplements are used for significant effects that cannot be attributed to single nutrients. To list just a few examples, such broad-range formulations have been documented to reduce inflammation,[13] increase muscular strength,[14] treat disease-related malnutrition,[15] increase cognitive performance in early Alzheimer's disease,[16] improve arterial stiffness,[17] and help in treatment in acute myocardial infarction,[18] hypertension, and cardiovascular disease.[19] The multinutrient approach can often be applied for both treatment and prevention.

MENTAL HEALTH TREATMENT THAT WORKS

Orthomolecular Medicine News Service, October 7, 2005

Doctors report that mental health problems including depression, bipolar disorder, schizophrenia, ADHD [attention deficit hyperactivity disorder], anti-social and learning disorders, and obsessive-compulsive disorders often have a common cause: insufficient nutrients in the brain. Nutritionally-oriented physicians assert that the cure for these problems is to give the body the extra nutrients it needs, especially when under abnormal stress.

Orthomolecular medical researchers say the future of psychiatry is in nutrition because nutrition has such a long, safe and effective history of correcting many mental problems. Nutrients such as the B vitamins are most successful when taken regularly, taken in relatively high doses, and taken in conjunction with vitamin C, the essential fatty acids (EFAs), and the minerals magnesium and selenium.

A summary of what has worked for many people follows below. The safety of vitamins and minerals is extraordinary, and the expense of trying them is much less than the cost of hazardous pharmaceutical drugs. These nutrients can be purchased in a discount or health store.

Taking 1,000 mg of vitamin B_3 three times a day often cures mild to moderate depression. Dramatic results are often achieved within one week of beginning this nutritional program, especially in alcoholics.[1]

Sometimes a simple deficiency of vitamin D causes depression. 3,000 IU/day from all sources can alleviate the problem.[2]

3,000 mg/day or more of niacin (vitamin B_3), along with the same quantity of vitamin C, taken in divided doses throughout the day can successfully treat both schizophrenia and bipolar disorder.[3]

Vitamins B_3, B_6, C and the minerals magnesium and zinc frequently produce a good response in ADHD and autistic children.[4]

Vitamins B_6, folate, and B_{12} taken together lower elevated homocysteine levels in the elderly while improving mental function.[5]

As pointed out by chemistry professor and vitamin discoverer Roger J. Williams, Ph.D.,[6] each individual has different nutritional needs and responds differently to nutrients. Are you tired of being depressed, suffering from anxiety, paying huge prescription drug bills for unsafe prescriptions that don't solve the problem or produce undesirable side effects? Are you tired of the piecemeal trial and error approach to finding a solution to your mental or emotional problems? If so, adults should consider the following nutritional protocol, which will bathe your brain and nerves in natural nutrients and may well produce dramatic results. The cost of trying the program below is less than the cost of a typical doctor's office visit. It is safe and convenient. All of these nutrients can be purchased at large discount stores.

After the morning meal take:

- A multivitamin tablet
- 1,000 mg of vitamin B$_3$ (as niacinamide or inositol hexanicotinate)
- One B-complex tablet
- 100 mg of vitamin B$_6$
- 1,200 mcg of vitamin B$_9$ (folate or folic acid)
- 1,000–2,000 IU of vitamin D (the lower number if you get sunshine, the higher number if you don't)
- 1,000 mg of vitamin C
- 200 mg of magnesium
- 50 mg of zinc
- 200 micrograms (mcg) of selenium
- 30 grams of soy protein powder and one tablespoon of lecithin granules mixed into a small glass of juice or milk, taken along with a supplement of omega-3 fatty acids [eicosapentaenoic acid (EPA), docosahexanoic acid (DHA), and alpha-linolenic acid (ALA)]

After the midday meal:

- 1,000 mg of vitamin B$_3$
- 1,200 mcg of folic acid
- 100 mg of vitamin B$_6$
- One B-complex tablet
- 1,000 mg of vitamin C
- 200 mg of magnesium

After the evening meal:

- A multivitamin tablet
- 1,000 mg of vitamin C
- 100 mg of vitamin B$_6$
- 1,000 mg of vitamin B$_3$
- One B-complex tablet

All of the above supplements are safe in the recommended amounts, as well as inexpensive and convenient. There is not even one death per year from vitamins. Pharmaceutical drugs, properly prescribed and taken as directed, kill over 100,000 Americans annually. Hospital errors kill still more.

Restoring health must be done nutritionally, not pharmacologically. All cells in all persons are made exclusively from what we drink and eat. Not one cell is made out of drugs.

The most common mistake made by people who take vitamins is they fail to take enough vitamins.

The reason one nutrient can cure so many different illnesses is because a deficiency of one nutrient can cause many different illnesses.

References

1. Hoffer, A. "Vitamin B₃: Niacin and Its Amide. DoctorYourself.com. http://www.doctoryourself.com/hoffer_niacin.html (accessed July 2012). Cheraskin, E., W. M. Ringsdorf, A. Brecher, A. *Psychodietetics: Food as the Key to Emotional Health.* New York: Bantam Books, 1974.

2. Vieth, R., S. Kimball, A. Hu, et al. "Randomized Comparison of the Effects of the Vitamin D₃ Adequate Intake Versus 100 mcg (4000 IU) per Day on Biochemical Responses and the Wellbeing of Patients." *Nutr J* 3(8) (Jul 19, 2004).

3. Hoffer, A. *Healing Schizophrenia: Complementary Vitamin & Drug Treatments.* Toronto: CCNM Press, 2004. Hawkins, D., L. Pauling. *Orthomolecular Psychiatry: Treatment of Schizophrenia.* San Francisco: W. H. Freeman, 1973. Hoffer A. *Niacin Therapy in Psychiatry.* Springfield, IL: Thomas, 1962.

4. Hoffer, A. *Healing Children's Attention and Behavior Disorders: Complementary Nutritional & Psychological Treatments.* Toronto: CCNM Press, 2004. Hoffer, A. *Dr. Hoffer's ABC of Natural Nutrition for Children: With Learning Disabilities, Behavioral Disorders, and Mental State Dysfunctions.* Kingston, ON: Quarry Press, 1999.

5. Selhub. J., P. F. Jacques, P. W. Wilson, et al. "Vitamin Status and Intake as Primary Determinants of Homocysteinemia in an Elderly Population." *JAMA* 270(22) (Dec 8, 1993):2693–2698. Verhoef, P., R. Meleady, L. E. Daly, et al. "Homocysteine, Vitamin Status and Risk of Vascular Disease." *Eur Heart J* 20(17) (Sep 1999):1234–1244.

6. Orthomolecular.org. "Mental Health Treatment That Works." Orthomolecular Medicine News Service, Oct 7, 2005. http://orthomolecular.org/resources/omns/v01n11.shtml (accessed August 2012).

Homeopathy

Neither of the authors are trained in homeopathic medicine. When it comes to homeopathic remedies, we think it is important to be open-minded but cautious. I (BHJ) remember Bill Walsh talking about three words you should avoid when talking to American doctors: orthomolecular, hair analysis, and homeopathy. Personally, we think there can be something to homeopathy, electromagnetic treatments, and other modalities of which we know much too little. However, homeopathy is very controversial. The importance of placebo in depression treatment studies is often quite significant. A review by Davidson found no placebo-controlled studies for homeopathy in depression.[20] However, a recent study by Adler from Brazil was not included in Davidson's review. This study claims to be the first RCT study of homeopathic treatment for depression that is not too small.[21] We recommend reviewing these two papers to help make an educated decision about this therapy.

CHAPTER 10

BIPOLAR DISORDER

"We are not ourselves When nature, being oppressed, commands the mind To suffer with the body."
—WILLIAM SHAKESPEARE (1564–1616) *KING LEAR*

Bipolar disorder poses serious risks, including life-threatening situations during episodes, so it is necessary to consult with a responsible physician experienced with this condition. Any changes in lifestyle or complementary treatments should be made with the physician's knowledge and cooperation.

WHAT IS BIPOLAR DISORDER?

Bipolar disorder (BD), formerly called manic-depressive illness, is an affective disorder in which one's mood swings between mania (extreme elevation of mood) and depression. It is divided into two types: Bipolar I, in which the patient has had at least one manic or mixed episode, and Bipolar II, in which there has been at least one major depressive and at least one hypomanic (mild manic) episode, but no manic or mixed episodes.

Genetic factors and their interaction with environment are important in BD. The increased use of antidepressant drugs is a triggering factor for manias or hypomanias. The most important medical drugs used for mood stabilizing in BD are lithium, antiepileptics, and neuroleptics (or antipsychotics). The mechanisms of lithium salts are still little known. One hypothesis is that Li^+ and Mg^{2+} compete for binding sites in the nervous system.[1]

BIPOLAR DISORDER AND WORSE

One readers writes:

I "lost" my mind in 1997 after my third child was born. In 1999 I was finally diagnosed with bipolar disorder and was put on lithium and Paxil. For the next two years I lived life from the couch with not enough energy to cook meals or respond to the children's needs. I cycled [through moods] every three days and dealt with almost constant horrible suicidal thoughts. There was a constant war going on in my head even though my body was made lethargic by the medications. My weight grew from 123 to 200 pounds until March of 2001, when I discovered nutritional therapy.

Originally I was interested in finding energy to be able to exercise to slow down or stop the weight gain, but to my surprise in addition to the energy I was hoping to find, my mental symptoms disappeared within just a few weeks of supplementing. I was then able to get off the medications that were making me lethargic, causing me to gain weight, and to not be able to care for my children or home.

I have my life back, and my children have their mother back. Of course my doctor thought of me as another "noncompliant" patient refusing to take her lithium. I feel very fortunate to have your research and that of others in your field to back up the "miraculous" healing that I experienced. It gives me much comfort and assurance that I am not the only one being helped so tremendously by megavitamin therapy . . . and that this is for real and not just a misperception on my part as my doctor would like for me to believe.

For the past nineteen months, my mind has been at peace. I've been able to work, and to homeschool my children. I have lost sixty of the eighty pounds I gained on medication. I have the energy and mental capability to cook, make and live by a budget, clean my home, cut my grass, and chauffeur the kids to church, scouts, the library, playgroups, etc. We also have been able to start a family home business which is successful.

Evolutionary View of Bipolar Disorder

With unipolar depression we can see there are evolutionary aspects of interest. There are similar perspectives in bipolar disorder as well. Animal research suggests that social rank relates to manic and depressive states.[2]

Affective disorders may be conceptualized as rhythm disorders. Disease expression is affected by daily and seasonal rhythms. Individuals with an affective sensitivity may get ill during a specific time of the year, and one of their symptoms is often a change in their daily rhythm. Most cells in the body have what are called "clock genes," and the governing clock genes are found in a brain area called *nucleus suprachiasmaticus*. The main factor affecting the circadian clock is sunlight. One hypothesis is that disruptions in the circadian clock underlie bipolar disorder.

Evolutionary origin of bipolar disorder (EOBD) is a hypothesis described by Julia A. Sherman. It emerges from ideas about the importance of the organism's biological clock and energy-regulating mechanism[3] and theories that BD descends from a pyknic (compact, cold-adapted body type) group.[4] The suggestion is that BD behaviors are highly derived adaptations to the selective pressures of extreme climatic conditions with long, severe winters and short summers.[5]

It may also have evolutionary implications that many bipolar patients and their relatives are comparatively creative people.[6]

DR. ABRAM HOFFER WRITES:

Marion, age thirty-two, consulted me October 2 because she suffered from chronic fatigue and was unable to cope with recurrent infections. She had been diagnosed bipolar psychosis (manic depressive) and had been on and off lithium for thirteen years. When on lithium her mood cycled very rapidly. In mid July she was diagnosed with depression and started on an antidepressant which was very helpful. But when I saw her she told me about the voices she had heard in the past, about her paranoia, poor memory, and difficulty with concentration. I started her on a dairy-free diet with ascorbic acid 1 gram after each meal, pyridoxine 250 mg daily, zinc citrate 50 mg daily, selenium 200 mcg daily, and a B complex 50 mgs once daily. By November 18 she was well. She had started to improve about ten days after starting on the program.

Orthomolecular Treatment of Bipolar Disorder

Single-nutrient studies of BD are limited in number. However, omega-3 fatty acids may reduce depressions in BD. This was first shown in a double-blind study by Andrew Stoll in 1999.[7] A meta-analysis of six interventions shows that adjunctive omega-3 may improve depressive symptoms in BD. However, it did not support omega-3 for mania.[8]

Folic acid at 200 micrograms (mcg) daily added to lithium reduced affective morbidity, especially in those with higher plasma folate.[9] The authors suggest 300–400 mcg folic acid would be useful in long-term lithium profylaxis.

N-acetylcysteine (NAC), 1 gram twice a day for twenty-four weeks, adjunctive to usual medication, reduced depression in BD patients.[10] NAC has neuroprotective properties and increases the important antioxidant glutathione.

For bipolar mania, positive results have been described for magnesium when added to verapamil, which is a calcium antagonist.[11] Magnesium and zinc act as modulators for the N-methyl-D-aspartate (NMDA) receptor.[12] The NDMA receptor is the predominant molecular device for controlling synaptic and memory function. Another target for these two minerals is GSK-3ß, a neural signaling pathway that is just one of several biochemical systems where lithium exerts its activity.[13]

In a study of current acute mania, 3 mg of folic acid was added to valproate.[14] After three weeks the group given folic acid had recovered significantly faster.

Reviews of combined treatments that included some nutrients[15] express an openness to integrated treatment. Difficult diseases require the consideration of all approaches, whichever works best.[16]

One of the most interesting findings is that bipolar disorder patients have mitochondrial dysfunctions.[17] Mitochondria are the powerhouses of the cell. In mitochondrial disorders the best treatment is a broad combination of nutrients.[18]

In 1999, while I was shopping with my wife, a man came up to me and greeted me as if he knew me. He told me I had seen him many years earlier and he added he had not had a drink in sixteen years. He was well and neatly dressed and buying groceries as my wife and I were. He was still taking 3 grams of niacin which he thought was great and we discussed the best way to take it. This morning I looked up his file. I first saw him in 1976 in the intensive care unit of the psychiatric hospital. He had suffered from mood swings all of his life. His diagnosis was chronic schizophrenia. He was admitted to a chronic mental hospital in 1970 following abuse of amphetamines. After that he was admitted to many hospitals. He suffered from hallucinations, voices and visions, paranoid ideas, mood swings, and was often hyperexcitable. He was very depressed. He had been in several fights, I considered him either suicidal or homicidal. He was admitted again in 1977 to another service and was not given any vitamins. Of course he had also been diagnosed bipolar. He drank a lot and used street drugs. After I saw him again I started him on niacin 1 gram after each meal, and ascorbic acid the same dose. I saw him last August 5, 1981. He had been abstinent for seventeen days. His response to niacin and ascorbic acid illustrates once more what can be achieved with chronic patients if they continue to remain on these vitamins for many years.

Orthomolecular Clinical Practice for Bipolar Disorder

Before researchers confirm the value of a new treatment, single clinicians have usually been on the right track for years or even decades. When Abram Hoffer started treating schizophrenic patients with niacin and ascorbate sixty years ago, he described it as a comparatively good treatment unless the patient had been ill for too many years. In time the treatment was broadened to include more nutrients and was also used for different disorders. However, relatively little was published on orthomolecular treatment of bipolar disorder. One reason for this is that Abram Hoffer defended an older concept of schizophrenia. He evaluated and treated as schizophrenia cases that by other psychiatrists were increasingly being diagnosed as bipolar disorder and borderline disturbance. Even if opinions differ on where to draw the line, many psychiatrists today agree that there is a continuum between schizophrenia and bipolar disorder, with an in-between syndrome called schizoaffective psychosis.[19]

Sometimes, new treatments have been discovered by patients themselves or their relatives far away from universities or industry. One example is the development of a broad-spectrum micronutrient supplement in southern Alberta, Canada. In 1994 Anthony Stephan's bipolar wife committed suicide as had her father sixteen years earlier. One year later two of his children were diagnosed with bipolar disorder type I, and conventional medication did not really help. Then Anthony met animal feed formulator David L. Hardy, who explained how nutritional supplementation programs helped pigs with behavior symptoms. The two men started to work with scientists and manufacturers to formulate a supplement for humans. Anthony's children responded to the formula, recovered, and were still healthy after discontinuing their medications. This supplement was later called EMPowerplus, and with time clinical research started.[20]

This multinutrient compound contains sixteen vitamins, fourteen minerals, three amino acids, and three antioxidants. Several open studies have been published on treating different psychiatric disorders with this formula, and overall the results have been promising. In a series of eleven cases with bipolar disorder the treatment was effective for mood stabilization and made a decrease of psychotropic medication possible.[21] A careful case study of a twelve-year boy with BD was successful,[22] and a database analysis with 358 bipolar disordered people showed that the supplement reduced symptom severity and the need for mood stabilizing medication.[23]

A General Perspective on Bipolar Treatment

Getting back to where this book started—about evolution and holism—regular sleep, food,[24] and a reasonable amount of physical and social activity is essential for coping with bipolar disorder. This is the basis of Interpersonal and Social Rhythm Therapy (IPSRT) which is applied as an adjunctive part of treatment for bipolar disorder.[25] IPSRT was developed by Professor Ellen Frank at the University of Pittsburgh School of Medicine. Even if this method can be seen as an important contribution to the integrative treatment of this difficult-to-treat disorder, IPSRT has not encompassed the necessity of specific nutrition. This is where orthomolecular medicine can make a difference.

PART THREE

NON-VITAMIN CURES FOR DEPRESSION

CHAPTER 11

IN THE NOW

"If we open a quarrel between the past and the present,
we shall find that we have lost the future."
—WINSTON CHURCHILL (1874–1965)

The problem with being depressed is that you really are. It is not an illusion; it is not because your thinking is "off." Depression is real. Some people are depressed simply because they are tired. The absence of sleep or the presence of children (the two often being linked) can stress and depress a person. Even a job you like can be stressful, and having to work a job you hate is certainly depressing. I (AWS) have been there. When I was twenty-three, my firstborn was seven months old and I was working on a dairy farm.

Herd of Cows?

Sure, I've heard of cows. I was partly responsible for operating a medium-security prison for cows. I milked over a hundred, twice a day, getting up at 3:30 A.M. and finishing around 7:00 P.M. I was tired all the time, never had enough money, and in constant danger every minute of my workday. If you do not believe that, I invite you to spend a few weeks trying it. Even very docile cows are really big. They are animals. If they get scared, they run. If you are in the way, you are toast. And that's with the *nice* ones. Not all cows are nice. I still remember, like it was yesterday, when Number 29 very deliberately kicked me full force, right on my wrist. Then there was that time when a huge, angry cow literally tried and darn near succeeded in climbing out *over* the steel bars in her milking stall, while I was below her attaching the milking machine to her belly. One day, a perfectly nice cow, in a hurry for grain, literally slammed my boss into the wall. Once I was caught by a hydraulic gate that crushed my abdomen, leading to necessary surgery for a hernia later in life. Even back then, in the late 1970s, I had already read *Be Here Now*, cover to cover, twice. But I was in a really crappy now, and if you have ever cleaned out a milking parlor, you know that I mean that literally. But that is where I was.

My day started long before dawn. Cows sleep remarkably soundly. And unlike horses, cows very much enjoy lying down, sleeping like big boulders in the night. And it was still night when I had to go out, find them in the field, wake them up, and entice tons of sleepy bovine to get their teats pinched by a milking machine. Thank heaven I did not have to milk any Black Angus. Good looking in daylight, invisible in the dark.

Once you get them inside, the work has just started. The morning milking took nearly five hours to do and you had to do it all over again at 3:00 P.M. Some of our cows' udders were nearly three feet wide. I know this because I am tall—wear a thirty-seven-inch sleeve—and I had to press the side of my head against a big cow's belly in order to reach across underneath her to attach the far-side teats to the milking machine. For some cows, my reach was barely adequate.

Oh, and another thing: When a cow urinates, it is time to back away, at least if you can. If they let it loose when you are below milking them, it is an even-money bet whether or not you can dodge the quarts of urine that come roaring out like a waterfall. If it's in the barn or the milk house, the cement floor results in a jeans-drenching splash that you have to see to fully appreciate.

The farm I worked at was overlooked by a community college handsomely sited on a nearby hill. Many a day I literally gazed up at that imposing educational complex and thought what one of the future Beatles had expressed when he saw his first rock and roll movie. Pointing to the screen, John Lennon said to his mates, "Now *that's* a good job."

Out the Barn Door

So, in flat depression desperation, I borrowed money and learned Transcendental Meditation. This is literally true: I did one of my first meditations in the feed barn, sitting atop a huge pile of hay. I know that sounds quaint if not downright romantic, but not really. I was alone—almost. As I meditated, I had a gentle touch of the St. Francis of Assisi experience. I heard and felt mice, here, there, and everywhere. Having thought the barn empty, or perhaps picking up on the good vibes, they came out, not of the woodwork but out of the haystack. They headed over my way having evidently called their friends. I sat there laughing because it was just so bizarre.

Meditation, for me, was a tremendous asset. It really helped, for all the obvious reasons that stress reduction helps. It also got me in touch with the real *me*. Result? I immediately looked for and found another job that was many miles away, literally and figuratively, from dairy farming. Ever since then, whenever I have been depressed at work, I have a never-fail motto: "It beats milking cows." Every job I have ever held since has been an improvement.

The biggest improvement of all was when I followed Mark Twain's example. As he said, "I hired a hall and gave a lecture. I have not done an honest day's work since." In other words, I continued my education and became an author and motivational speaker. In between working so hard then and not having a *real* job at all now, I experienced what I think is a lovely irony: About fifteen years ago, I somehow ended up teaching at the very college that I previously looked up at from the dairy barnyard. My laboratory classroom literally looked out over the cornfield where I went out to pick some lunch and eat it raw off the cob. I would have my students go over to the window, and I'd point out to them just where I'd worked my agricultural tail off all those years ago. I do not in any way mean to demean farming. It is good, honest, hard work, and I told my students exactly that. Then I told them my hours, chores, and pay. I think I had the best stay-in-school lecture in academia.

When students asked Professor Joseph Campbell for life advice, he told them, "Follow your bliss." Surely this applies to depression.

First, you need to find what your bliss isn't, and that's a snap. Being depressed is nobody's bliss. That's a good start. The Chinese have said for millennia, "When you are sick of sickness, you are no longer sick."

Depression is universal. Centuries ago, the Buddha famously taught: There is suffering. There is a cause to suffering. There is an end to suffering. There is a path that puts an end to suffering. These remain the four noble truths of Buddhism. The first one is the kicker. Denying that you are suffering does not work. Telling someone to "cheer up!" does not work. When you are depressed, and just about everyone has been, accepting that reality is a necessary start.

Most books, therapists, and advice-proffering friends tend to move too quickly right along to truths two, three and four. They want to find out what's eating you, tell you that everything will be all right, and coach you out of it. All of this is well intended, compassionate, and often helpful. After all, when you are the one in the bag, it is hard to see outside of the bag. Diagnosis, encouragement, and treatment are understandable responses. This book does a good bit of that as well.

But again, let's return to truth one: There is depression, and you have it. You really feel the way you do, right here, right now.

There is something good in that bald realization. Being right here, right now, is in itself a way out of depression.

"Wait a minute. I'm *depressed* in the here and now. How does it help me to be even more in the very here and now that is so rotten?"

Being Here Now

An insightful, remarkably practical answer is provided by *The Power of Now,* by Eckert Tolle. The main point in Tolle's teaching is deceptively simple: remain conscious that you are in the now. Dr. Richard Alpert (also known as Ram Dass) said the same thing decades ago, in his book *Be Here Now.*

You do not have to look outside the Christian faith for such a message. Jesus said, "And which of you by being anxious can add one cubit unto the measure of his life?" (Matthew 6:27) "Be not therefore

THE POWER OF NOW BY ECKHART TOLLE,

Reviewed by John I. Mosher, Ph.D.,
Biology Professor Emeritus, State University of New York

After years of mental anguish, suffering much as most of us have, Eckhart Tolle has written The *Power of Now*. His book is a presentation of age-old truths with a transformative insight, delivered in a manner to which those of us from the western industrial, materialistic culture can easily relate. As with a sword, Mr. Tolle cuts through the confusion of our personal, and national, suffering and offers insights into the basis of that suffering. The domination of the ego-mind consciousness seems to be the culprit. On pages 130–131, Mr. Tolle comments on interpersonal relationships as an example:

"As humans have become increasingly identified with their mind, most relationships are not rooted in BEING and so turn into a source of pain and become dominated by problems and conflict. . .

"The opportunity that is concealed within every crisis does not manifest until all the facts of any given situation are acknowledged and fully accepted. As long as you deny them, as long as you try to escape from them or wish that things were different, the window of opportunity does not open up, and you remain trapped inside that situation, which will remain the same or deteriorate further."

But wait: things are not hopeless. According to Mr. Tolle, you can create a place in your consciousness for transformation. You can begin to heal yourself from the inside out. Again quoting the author:

"When you know you are not at peace, your knowing creates a still space that surrounds your nonpeace in a loving and tender embrace and then transmutes your nonpeace into peace. As far as inner transformation is concerned, there is nothing you can do about it. You cannot transform yourself, and you certainly cannot transform your partner or anybody else. All you can do is create a space for transformation to happen, for grace and love to enter."

How do you "create a space for transformation to happen"? By mindfulness, prayer, meditation, and practicing positive states of mind. By practicing positive states of mind such as compassion, tolerance, selflessness, and love. By following practices which calm and stabilize the mind, practicing positive states of mind, observing when you are thinking (i.e. strengthening your ability to witness your own thoughts and actions) so that you can choose not to give power to a troubling situation. Feeling your internal energy fields the mind a rest and brings more power to your essential Self, which is the reality of who you *really* are. As your true essence becomes more dominant and the thinking mind is used only as a tool or servant to you, then peace, unconditional love, happiness, and transformation begin to take place. The secret is to go within. This is what spiritual practice, stress-reducing practices, and practices that calm and stabilize the mind, are ideally intended to do. From my understanding of Mr. Tolle's message, this is a way for practicing *The Power of Now.*

I highly recommend *The Power of Now,* and Mr. Tolle's other book, *Practicing the Power of Now,* as guides for your journey to enjoying good health, long life, and happiness.

Reprinted with permission of the author and DoctorYourself.com (http://www.doctoryourself.com/nowpower.html).

anxious for the morrow: for the morrow will be anxious for itself. Sufficient unto the day is the evil thereof." (Matthew 6:34) "No man, having put his hand to the plow, and looking back, is fit for the kingdom of God." (Luke 9:62) These are all "now" statements.

It has been said that if something is true, wherever you look, you will find it. One thing that is absolute in life is that the past is gone forever (*Time Tunnel* reruns notwithstanding). Another absolute is that the future is utterly unknown. That pretty much leaves us with the present . . . and nothing but the present. Appropriately, that is the focus of the writings of both Ram Dass and Eckert Tolle. The inner peace and corollary benefits to practicing being really here, really now, need to be experienced by you, directly for yourself. No one can do it for you: you are the C.E.O. of Y.O.U.

Some of this we've surely heard before, and even if we agree, it is not enough. You cannot force it by putting on a happy face and straining to smile. If you are down, then you are. Acknowledge that. It's here, it's true, it's real, and it's you. *For now.*

Since my farm days, meditation notwithstanding, I have had my full share of times of diagnosable depression. Once I was very severely, terribly depressed. I remember the absolute hour and day I bottomed out. It was the very black pit of despair. Usually I have always been able to quickly find at least ten things in my life to be thankful for. (Truth be told, there are probably thousands.) But at that bleak moment, I could literally find only five. I was alive; I had a roof over my head; I was not starving; I was not sick or injured; I still had a few friends and living relatives. That was it. Everything else was a catastrophic mess. It was worse than living out the worst country-western song.

With the benefit of hindsight, I can tell you that it helped me immensely to simply see myself sitting there, miserable and without a glimmer of hope or a speck of initiative. I saw *Me* experiencing it for what it was, right there, right now.

Well goody, you might be thinking. There I am. I see myself, and Me is damned depressed. How exactly does that change things?

Here's the trick: *If you are seeing yourself depressed, who is doing the seeing?*

Eureka! The real *You* is seeing you. Because this is a book, I capitalized the real You. The other "you" is still you. No, this is not a license to carry a concealed split personality. It is a solid technique that really works.

Here it is again: See yourself depressed. There I am. Man, I am miserable. Look at me there. Just look at me! Have you ever seen such anguish? Yep, that's me all right, and Me is hurting bad.

Now who is doing the seeing? That is the inner, timeless part of You that is doing the seeing. That You is not depressed. It was always there, always here. As my favorite Zen saying goes, you have been riding around on the ox searching for that ox.

But What if This Does Not Work?

Perhaps the greatest contribution Eckert Tolle has made to this approach is this: If you have difficulty being in the now, notice yourself having difficulty being in the now. If you notice yourself having difficulty in the now, you are automatically in the now. You are seeing yourself not being in the now, so you are in the now.

This is not just wordplay, and it is not pop psychology. It is a two-step plan that anyone can do, anywhere, anytime. It costs nothing and it has no adverse side effects. And, it works.

Once again: be here now. If you can't, if your mind is racing or your heart is broken, or your hopes are dashed, see yourself experiencing that. Be here now. That's you. See yourself?

Then who is doing the seeing?

And remember Tolle's failsafe backup plan. If you simply cannot be in the now, then acknowledge it and notice yourself *not* being in the now. The moment you do so, you are automatically in the now. "Yep, that's me. I'm off again. See? I am not even close to being in the now. I'm pining over the past and fretting about the future. Am I in the now? No way."

Right. So then who is making these observations? That is the part of you that is in the now.

Following the *be in the now* technique will help you reach inside and see who You really are, right here, right now.

The next chapter specifically sets out what you can do next.

CHAPTER 12

UNSTRESS AND UN-DEPRESS YOUR LIFE

by John I. Mosher, Ph.D.

*"If you change yourself you will change your world.
If you change how you think then you will change how
you feel and what actions you take. And so
the world around you will change."*

—MOHANDAS KARAMCHAND GANDHI
(MAHATMA GANDHI) (1869–1948)

THE BARROOM FIGHT

I used to startle my students by saying, "Do you know why I never get into barroom fights? Well, the reason is very simple, it is because I don't go into barrooms." The point I was making with this comment is, if you don't go there, it cannot happen!

A lot of a person's suffering comes from going to a place, either physically or mentally, that causes suffering to them. A goodly amount of our suffering or stressful discomfort amounts to choices we make and perhaps creative solutions we do not make. So the obvious lesson to be learned and acted upon is to make choices which are most likely to reduce the stress and promote wellbeing. That is, make choices when possible to avoid stressful situations.

Many times we do not have a choice. For example if your job is stressful and you like the job or are unable to change jobs then another

149

strategy must be used. When one is unable to change the physical circumstances then one's perception must be altered. In her classic book,
Eleanor H. Porter has the heroine, Pollyanna, doing this all the time.
The technique Pollyanna uses to view what might be an unpleasant
or stressful situation in a positive way is sometimes called "The Glad
Game." Pollyanna plays the "Glad Game" by viewing all situations
in a positive way. She tries to find what she can be glad about in the
situation. By seeing the positive aspects of a situation you may turn
that situation from an unpleasant or stressful one into a challenge or
some kind of learning experience. For example I think there is general
agreement that the emotion of anger is quite stressful.

I was talking with a woman one day and she made the comment
that when things did not go as she hoped she got angry. I thought to
myself: she must be angry quite a lot. It does not seem like a very creative way to approach the problems inherent in life. I said to her, "You
mean you would get angry if you went to use your car and found a tire
was flat?"

"Yes, that would really make me mad: one more thing to contend
with!" she responded.

Then I said, "Well, after you were upset and put your nervous system through all the stress of being angry what would you have to do?"

"I guess I would have to get the tire repaired or replaced," she said.

I then suggested to her that she might like to try a new approach for
getting her tire fixed which leaves out the anger. I said, "Why not try
a three step approach?"

1. **Observe** the flat tire.

2. **Accept** the fact that it needs to be repaired or replaced.

3. **Act** and get the tire replaced or repaired.

By accepting the situation as it is, it leaves one free to do what is
necessary to remedy that particular situation. By using the approach of
accepting the situation, stress and anger is eliminated. Of course such
a situation may be inconvenient and cause expense, but that is how it
is. So we work with how it is.

Two weeks later I saw the woman and she said, "Guess what, the brakes on my car failed, I started to get angry, then I remembered our conversation and I carefully proceeded to a garage and got the brakes fixed. Yes, I wished that it had not happened, it was inconvenient, but I accepted the situation and took the necessary action. That was the end of it and I felt much better and more in charge, and that I had learned a way to reduce the emotional stress of getting angry every time things did not go as I wished."

By reminding herself that it was not necessary to get angry, she accepted the situation without anger and just got the car repaired. This type of perceptual change in one's view of an undesirable circumstance may eliminate a lot of stress. It is also more efficient to go right to acceptance and then problem solving, leaving out the emotional reaction.

In the case of a mental or emotional situation such as the loss of a job or the break-up of a relationship the same approach may apply. Like the barroom fight, if you don't go there it cannot happen. So in the case of an emotional situation, the mind tends to go there and to obsess about the situation.

The powerful feelings of rejection are very hard on one's self image, especially if one's self-image depends on externals such as always having the approval of others. The loss of a job or the loss of a relationship, again, are just life situations, in many ways not unlike the flat tire, except they involve more of the mind-created identity called ego and the thinking mind. If you allow your attention to go to this place, the place of attachment, fear, and regret, certainly you will suffer. However, if you recognize your feelings, without dwelling on them or denying them, you are positioned for a new step.

The new step is to accept the situation as it is and then move your attention within, that is, within the body in general. Do not allow your attention to go to the thinking mind. Be present in the moment of feeling your internal life energy. By going to the place of your body's life energy, you are not obsessing about your life situation. By staying in the place of your life which is right here, right now, you are not replaying in your mind the "would have been, could have been, should have been" scenario. Instead, what you are doing is accepting the situation. You are staying conscious by recognizing and accepting the situation and realizing that no amount of obsessing thoughts or regrets will help. What *will* help is moving on to the present, the right here, right now, the only place you are really alive. As painful as the occurrence may have been, it does not help you to go over it except to consider what you learned from the experience. If you lost your job because you were consistently late for work then learn you must be punctual. If you lost your relationship because you were not dependable, then realize the importance of keeping your word. In general, after you have looked over the situation and gleaned the teaching, accept it and get on with your life by staying in the present. Deal with the here and now, and do not go to the place of the obsessing mind. I am not suggesting denial.

You do not deny. You recognize your feelings, then accept the situation, then do what is appropriate. It is always good to keep your consciousness in the present. The reality of life is that all you ever really have is the "now," the present. There is a Native American saying which illustrates this: "Yesterday is ashes, tomorrow is wood, only today does the fire burn brightly."

> Take time to think about why you do what you do, why you feel what you feel, why you see life the way you do.
> Does your way of seeing, feeling, and doing bring happiness to you and those around you?
> What is your dream?

Avoid barroom fights by avoiding barrooms. Physically you can make choices to avoid stressful places. Mentally you can avoid stressful places by accepting the situation, taking appropriate measures and staying present. By practicing the relaxation exercises described below, you are practicing being present. Be mindful of going within. Going within can simply mean putting your attention on your natural breathing rhythm. Practice this: at every opportunity go within; be mindful. Be aware of your breath; be aware of the energy in your body; feel the awareness of being. Be sure you are breathing diaphragmatically. Stay mindful of the life force within.

Here's how to start:

GETTING STARTED IMMEDIATELY

Practicing stress reduction is like a breath of cool mountain air; like the refreshing water of a quiet lake shore among the silent pines. Here in this peaceful sanctuary, you feel your own being as the quiet still point within. Come to this quiet peaceful place. Even in the midst of the toil and turmoil of the day, find peace. Let's help you commence that metaphorical "breath of cool mountain air."

Summary of a Relaxation Technique

1. Have a quiet, comfortable place to do your practice.

2. Close your eyes and breathe from your diaphragm for a few seconds or longer to establish diaphragmatic breathing.

3. With eyes closed, coordinate the position of your tongue with the inhale and the exhale (as explained in the detailed instructions, below). Repeat this procedure at least three times. You may do more if you wish.

4. With eyes closed, do the alternating breathing (as described below). Be sure you breathe from the diaphragm. Do this type of breathing for about five minutes.

5. With eyes closed, do mindful diaphragmatic breathing for fifteen to twenty minutes.

6. At the end of the fifteen or twenty minutes of "mindful" breathing, rest with eyes closed for at least five minutes. After the rest, commence activity gradually. Be gentle with yourself!

Practice the technique, as instructed, twice a day, once before eating in the morning and before the evening meal. You may do a short ten-minute session before your noon meal if you wish. Remember, something is better than nothing. If you cannot organize your time to include two sessions per day, do one. Of course, two a day gives results more quickly, and naturally is more effective.

Remember you can go as slowly or as quickly on this program as you wish.

HOW TO PROCEED

Choose a quiet comfortable place. It is best to do the procedure sitting up with the back comfortably straight.

With eyes closed, be aware of your breathing. Be sure you are breathing from the diaphragm, not the chest. That is, when breathing, your lower abdominal area should rise and fall noticeably with your inhale and exhale. There should be only minimal movement of the chest.

Once you have established proper diaphragmatic breathing with your eyes closed, then try coordinating your tongue position with the inhale and exhale like this:

Put your tongue on the roof of your mouth just behind your upper front teeth, with your mouth closed on the inhale. Inhale fully in this position. Hold your breath to the count of seven, then drop your tongue to its normal position on the floor of your mouth. Open your mouth slightly and slowly exhale. When exhalation is complete, hold your breath to the count of seven and then close your mouth, place your tongue on the roof of your mouth, and inhale. Repeat this form of breathing three times (more if you wish). Remember keep your eyes closed and keep your awareness on your breathing.

After having completed three or more breaths as described above, proceed, with eyes closed, to alternating breathing.

The alternating breathing consists of (a) Breathing normally from the diaphragm, (b) using your thumb to close your right nostril, inhaling through the left nostril. Next, release the right nostril and close the left nostril with your fingers and exhale through the right nostril. Then inhale through the right nostril. Close the right nostril with your thumb and exhale through the left nostril, then inhale through the left nostril, close and exhale through the right nostril. Continue the alternating nostrils breathing for five minutes with your eyes closed.

Now discontinue the alternating breathing technique. As you continue to sit quietly with your eyes closed, bring your attention to your breath. Continue to breathe from the diaphragm.

Be mindful of inhaling and exhaling. If you wish, you may think the word "SO" as you inhale and the word "HUM" as you exhale.

Continue this "mindful" breathing for fifteen or twenty minutes. If during breathing your mind wanders and gets off on thoughts, simply turn your attention from the thought back to the breathing as soon as you realize that your attention is not on breathing but on thoughts. Do not try to control your thoughts; do not dwell on them. Just let the thoughts pass by as a stream would flow past you. If you realize that your mind is on thoughts and not mindful of the breathing again, turn your attention from the thoughts back to the breathing.

At the end of fifteen or twenty minutes of the mindful breathing lie down and relax with your eyes closed for at least five minutes. At the end of your rest commence with activity nice and slowly. Avoid any immediate strenuous activity. Even though your mind may seem very alert, remember that you body has been at profound rest. It would sort of jolt the body to immediately jump up from your rest and start strenuous activity. Be gentle and easy with your body.

Remember: try to practice this technique twice a day: morning before eating and evening before eating. If you wish you may do a five or ten minute session before eating lunch.

Feel the Life in Your Own Body

With your eyes closed and breathing at the diaphragm level, bring your attention to your feet and ankles. Notice them, give them your attention! How do they feel? Just allow your attention to be there. If there is any sensation, such as discomfort, just allow your attention to be there.

When you are ready, proceed in the same manner with your mind's eye, your observer, to survey and feel each part of your body. Starting as described with the feet and ankles, move up the legs, hips, lower back, abdomen, chest, hands, arms, shoulders, neck, jaw, face, and the crown of the head. If there is any sensation of whatever nature in any area, allow yourself to experience it for as long as you wish. Then move on. If you feel adventurous (and anatomically savvy), you may extend this survey to your internal organs as well, such as the intestines, kidneys, liver, stomach, lungs, heart, and so on. As you do this just let your attention be with the area you are surveying for a moment or two or as long as you wish.

If there is discomfort at any area of your body that you are survey-ing then allow your attention to remain on that area. You may notice, at first, that this discomfort becomes more obvious when you first pay attention to it; that is normal. You will notice that after a short period of intense discomfort that the feeling will seem to disappear. The area under surveillance will just feel neutral. At this point move on to the next area.

Moving Your Body

A light exercise program is always helpful to the mind and body. Much has been written about the value of massage, stretches, yoga asanas (positions), T'ai Chi, and various other light exercises. Traditionally, some sort of stretches or postures with a self-massage are suggested before doing a relaxation or meditative practice. Yes, you can give yourself a massage. Start with the head. Massage your scalp and then continue to the forehead, the temples, around the eyes, your cheeks, and jaws. Then massage the back of your neck and continue on to your throat. Be very gentle with the throat area.

Massage your throat on either side of the windpipe with your finger tips. Then continue down the neck to the shoulders. The hands and wrists are next. Massage your hands like you are washing them, and proceed to the wrists and on up your arm. After doing each arm start at the waist and massage as much of your back as you can. Upon com-pleting the back, massage the lower abdomen working your way up to the chest area. Next start with your feet and work your way up your leg to the waist. After completing the self massage start progressively tensing and relaxing the muscles of your feet, then your calves, then your thighs, buttocks, arms, shoulders, and any other muscles around the waist, back, and chest area that you are able to tense and relax. Move on to your face and tense and relax your jaws and other face muscles as best you can.

If you wish a more extensive pre-relaxation body movement you might join a yoga class or get a book outlining various movements, yoga postures, and stretches. It is up to you as to how much you wish to include. If you have time and inclination, of course it is beneficial to do as much as possible. But if your time is limited, then at least start with just the self massage. Light exercise in general is very good to help reduce stress. A walk in the fresh air along a beach or stream, or in a park or woods, can be very invigorating and beneficial. If you are not already including a fifteen minute or more walk in your daily life, it is time to do so.

During the day, either at home or at work, take a minute or two just to stretch and tense and relax your muscles. Even if you are traveling, you can tense and relax your muscles while you are seated.

A woman upon celebrating her 100th birthday was, predictably, asked for the secret for longevity.
She stated that she thought that not worrying was a major factor in extending her life.
"I discovered," she said, "that 95 percent of what I worried about when I was young never happened, and that the small percent of what did happen was beyond my control. So, I realized that worrying was a waste of time and mental energy. From then on I trained myself not to worry."

Being Present

Throughout your normal day, wherever you are, try this: be present, and be right where you are, right now. Thoughts, especially negative thoughts, tend to take you away from the present. They may move you back to the past where you may have sadness, regrets, or grief. Or, you may have anxious thoughts of the future, which of course has not happened yet. But those thoughts are about the past or the future, not the present. Just take a moment to realize that the past is gone and the future has not happened. You are only living right this moment. So, to live in the present means to be right here, right now—not in the past nor in the future. This idea is very difficult for some to grasp because their mind is always dwelling in the past or flitting ahead to the future. So begin by considering that you are right here, right now, and not in the past nor in the future.

During the day actively seek thoughts. You might start by closing your eyes a second or two and ask yourself, "I wonder what my next thought will be?" Watch for the thought as you might watch a fox den to see if a fox will come out. If a fox—that is, a thought—comes out, observe it and let it go. This shows you that you can observe thoughts and make choices. If thoughts try to dominate your awareness, remind yourself that You are in charge. As the observer of thoughts you can say that "the thoughts are obsessing and I do not need to pay any attention to them." When thoughts take over, you lose consciousness. Every time you realize that you are thinking about the past or the future, bring your attention back to the observer stage. That is the observer watching and making choices. The observer who can choose to be right here, right now. As you practice this technique of observing your thoughts and letting them pass, you will live more in the present. You will have more consciousness and be able to make choices rather than responding in a reflexive way to thoughts. Remember, thoughts are just thoughts and they do not have to be acted upon. Thoughts may be observed like watching fallen leaves drift by on the surface of a stream. You do not have to do anything; just watch them go by. Practice this concept during your daytime activity. It may be difficult at first. Thoughts will want to take over and dominate. It takes time, and practice.

Irritant or Pearl?

There are perceptions and outlooks on life's situations that can turn what appears to be an uncomfortable, undesirable, or stressful situation into one of gain. An example of this would be the pearl. The beautiful, desirable pearl has a beginning that, to the oyster, may seem like an unpleasant situation. A grain of sand that gets inside the oyster's shell is an irritant. This ongoing irritation causes the oyster to form a smooth protective coating around the irritating sand. This coating eventually becomes the pearl. If the oyster can do it, why can't we? Why can't we take the obvious, the irritant, the stressful situation, and reverse it to produce a pearl of great wisdom or at least a positive situation?

Reacting to a stress with frustration and anger just produces more stress. But if you take the situation and keep your awareness, you may reverse the obvious and bring compassion, tolerance, forgiveness, and understanding to the situation. Therefore, instead of taking the low-road response of adding more anger or chaos to the situation, you have reversed it by bringing calmness and peace to the situation. A simple example of how this idea might be brought into an ordinary frustrating situation is one of misplaced keys. You may be in a great hurry and discover you cannot find your car keys. One obvious response would be to get upset and blame others, and storm around shouting and raging. This behavior does not find your keys, and may actually be so distracting that it hinders you from systematically looking for your keys. It may even cloud your perception and keep you from remembering where you may have put them. This behavior or irritation will be repeated endlessly until you observe that this behavior does not solve the problem of misplacing your keys. When the light of realization finally goes on, your internal observer, the Knower, might say, "This will always happen until you make a change." The change to be made is simple: just develop the habit of always leaving your keys in the same place. This simple change solves the problem.

From the irritating, inconvenient situation comes the motivation to change. I believe the purpose of much of the irritation, pain, and suffering in our life situation is really to function as a stimulus to get our attention, to wake-up and change! Perhaps taking the obvious negative experience and reversing it or transforming it into a positive life-supporting situation is the ultimate challenge.

The pearls of wisdom, such as the recognition of beauty, love, and happiness, can arise from a seemingly demanding, unpleasant situation. With discipline, some creative thinking, and practice we can create "pearls" out of what may seem to be distressing and undesirable.

How to Practice Mindfulness

Mindfulness is rooted in both Buddhist tradition and evolutionary psychology. Used as a complementary treatment for depression, it has been shown to have a modest effect both for treatment and relapse prevention of depression.[1]

A major part of stress reduction is learning to be mindful. That means to be aware and conscious of your thoughts and what you are doing. For example, let's say you are standing in line at the cashier of a grocery store and having negative and impatient thoughts. First, realize that you are having these thoughts. When you do, immediately make the choice to observe the thoughts, be aware of them, and let them go. Replace the space with positive thoughts. You might think "I wish all the people in line and in the store happiness, good health, and success." Actually send thoughts of love and appreciation to them, and especially to the cashier who is working so fast to reduce the size of the line. Put yourself in her or his place and send them kind thoughts. So by practicing or cultivating positive states of mind you are putting uplifting intentions into the surroundings. Practice the technique of being present and consciously replacing negative thoughts and feelings with ones of compassion, selflessness, tolerance, kindness, forgiveness, gratitude, and appreciation. This is a good start to reducing much stress. Remind yourself that there is no written rule that says things have to be the way you think they should be. Take a life situation as it is and bring as much love and compassion into it as you can.

Over and over again, research results point out that a positive attitude toward life, a sense of humor, and laughter strengthen the immune system and even seem to extend one's life. Be present, and think positively!

Get Away from It All

Go to a peaceful place as often as you can. A relatively easy way to do this is to practice the techniques that have been outlined in this chapter. All these techniques can, in a real sense, provide you with a portable sanctuary: a sanctuary where you can go within and be with your Being, that still point within, in almost any place or any time of your choosing. Having said that, I encourage you to create a special sacred place to use for just being with yourself. Joseph Campbell writes: "This is a place where you can simply experience and bring forth what you are and what you might be. This is the place of creative incubation. At first you might find that nothing happens there. But if you have a sacred place and use it, something eventually will happen . . . your sacred space is where you find yourself again and again."

I also like to make sacred physical spaces out of doors. I created such a space in the rather secluded southwest corner of our lawn. I also have a space in a friend's nearby woods. I completely agree with Henry David Thoreau when he wrote, "I went to the woods because I wished to live deliberately, to front only the essential facts of life, and see if I could not learn what it had to teach and not when I came to die, discover that I had not lived."

Being in nature and enjoying beautiful, quiet landscape is healing. A lot of our illness, both physical and mental, comes from our disconnection from the natural world. I knew a young man years ago who was afraid to be alone in the woods. His fear in general was so profound that he felt physically debilitated in certain ways when in a strange natural setting. To my way of thinking, this situation signaled the depth of his disconnection not only from nature, but from his true natural self. The mind and mind-created ego were so powerful, through his mental conditioning from home, education, and society in general, that he seemed out of touch with his true being. I was more fortunate. As a boy growing up on a farm, I loved to ramble in the fields, hedgerows, woods, and streams. I enjoyed seeing what was going on out of doors. There always seemed to be some activity, be it bird, insect, deer, woodchuck, field mouse, or snake. All were just being and following their natural patterns of life. Just being away from people and with the wild plants and animals was a balancing and comforting experience for me. Over the years, without consciously realizing it, I used the time in the out-of-doors as a stress management program. Fortunately my studies, research, and teaching in the biological sciences required quite a lot of time spent out of doors. I think one of my major experiences in finding myself occurred when I was studying big horn sheep in an unmapped wilderness area in southwestern Colorado. I was camped near the snow, which covered the mountain top. It was July, and I was at about 12,000 feet above sea level. I could see forever, so it seemed, and my only contact with the populated world was the glint of sun from a metal roof on a ranch about twenty or more miles away. I was alone and the only sounds were those of nature. Absolutely no human signs: just animal tracks and pathways.

In my early adult years, with the pressures of career and family, the woods were my salvation. I had the feeling that there were ways of gaining that benefit of nature when it was not possible to be out in the woods. Deep within me I knew there must be a way to live that was not so stressful. I remember thinking that there must be more to life than the everyday pressures and the treadmill of ego-gratifying accomplishments in the name of career and science. My reflective quiet time in the woods felt settling and gratifying, unlike my career accomplishments. It seemed that regardless of what one might achieve at the job or in the field of research, the satisfaction from the accomplishment soon faded. It was somewhat like being addicted to a substance: there is the short-term high but no long-term liberation from the peaks and valleys of the cycle. What I wanted was a stable, permanent happiness. At this point I realized that pleasure is a short term, transitory experience, whereas happiness is a basic underlying positive attitude toward life. This involves cultivating the positive values of life such as compassion, selflessness, tolerance, forgiveness, and kindness, along with having gratitude and appreciation for one's own life as well as that of others. I found that adopting and practicing these values takes self discipline and the need to remain mindful and conscious of one's life situation. For example, if someone is unpleasant to you, your initial reaction may be one of anger. But by remaining conscious, you can acknowledge your feeling and then make a conscious choice not to act on the feeling. You can use this life situation to realize that happy people do not act unpleasantly. The unpleasant person surely is in pain. There is an old saying that the amount of pain one inflicts on another is directly proportional to the amount of pain they feel inside.

Realizing the possibility that the other is unpleasant because they are in pain allows you to practice compassion. Then, instead of yelling or punching the person, you can say, "I'm sorry you feel that way." By doing this you have remained conscious and perhaps even helped the other person to examine their own motivations. At the very least you have helped yourself, and at the most you have been compassionate and understanding to another person, giving them the opportunity to grow in their own realization.

Spending time in your sanctuary, be it a room, a park, a wood, or a mountain top, gives you the opportunity and the peace to put things in perspective. Just being in nature and allowing the noise and chatter of the mind to be somewhat neutralized by the silence of the trees is beneficial. If you have the privacy of a wood available, you might try letting yourself be drawn to a certain tree. Go to that tree and lean against it, with your forehead and hands touching the tree. As you spend a minute or two or more doing this, you will note a peaceful feeling coming over you. You may even feel that you are experiencing your surroundings differently than you usually do. It has been said that trees function as a great antenna, bringing in the coherent energy of the cosmos. Perhaps the tree tunes up your nervous system; who can say? Regardless of theory, the fact is that many others, as well as myself, have experienced healing and feelings of well-being from such contact.

We are stressed and restless, always looking for something outside of ourselves to make us happy. The techniques, the sanctuary, the practice of cultivating positive states of mind all facilitate our discovering ourselves again and again until we are enjoying living.

(Reprinted with permission of the author.)

CHAPTER 13

DEPRESSION: OBSERVATIONS AND COMMENTS

by John I. Mosher, Ph.D.

Depression," "The Blues," "Feeling Down," "Feeling Sad" are all titles that have been given to an uncomfortable feeling of hopelessness and despair. It does not matter what one calls that feeling, but what does matter is to get relief from that feeling. To transition to a feeling of hopefulness, optimism, happiness, and generally a feeling of well being is facilitated by taking responsibility for your health.

There is a saying that "a problem cannot be solved at the level of the problem." Some new element has to be introduced to the problematical situation. For example, if the problem is darkness in a room, studying all about darkness does not solve the problem. However, when the new element of light is introduced the darkness vanishes and the problem of darkness is solved. Would this approach work in solving the problem of depression? Yes, research has shown that many cases have been helped by introducing a new element. A few of these new elements include good nutrition, nutritional supplements, meditation, positive affirmation, and counseling. It seems that these elements help transform the negative obsessive thought loops.

Dr. Jill Bolte Taylor, a brain scientist, has worked with the process of balancing and modifying unwanted thought "loops."[1] She emphasizes being vigilant of negative thoughts and noting any physiological body reactions that accompany those thoughts. This being done, steps are then taken to modify feelings and reactions by talking to the brain

165

to correct the negative thinking. According to Dr. Taylor there seems to be a group of brain cells that tap into our negative attitudes of jealousy, fear, and rage. These cells in our verbal mind are resourceful in their ability to run our thinking loops of doom and gloom. They thrive when they are generally being negative, complaining, and viewing how awful everything is. These cells seem to feed on negativity. This feeding on negativity reminds me of the story of the good wolf and the bad wolf. The wolf that will thrive is the one that is fed. So let's feed the good wolf that represents the cells with the joyful positive outlook. It is Dr. Taylor's belief that over 99 percent of cells in (her) brain and body want her to be happy, healthy, and successful. Considering her belief and the wolf story, it is obvious that we need to feed not just the 99 percent but 100 percent of our cells with the essential raw materials of nutrition and positive practices and behaviors such as meditation and affirmations.

Therefore the problem of depression is modified in a positive way by introducing the elements supporting good nutrition and the elements facilitating a positive emotional environment in the individual.

If a person suffering from depression consulted me, the first thing I would suggest is that they take responsibility and be proactive in investigating a holistic approach to finding balance.

Specifically I would suggest to them the following bare-bones strategy to aid them on their journey of restoring harmony and balance in their lives:

1. **See yourself as being in charge, take responsibility.** *Let go of the victim role!*

2. **Consult with a holistic orthomolecular health care practitioner who is experienced in treating depression.** Review your eating habits, correct them if necessary, and supplement as directed by your practitioner.

3. **Address the voices in your head that are telling you negative stories.** Try to envision a body with these voices. Make the body look ridiculous so you would not listen to such a ridiculous looking clown. Tell the voices to go back to their source; that there is no place for

them with you. These voices may be coming from the brain cells that Dr. Taylor alludes to as the ones running thinking loops of doom and gloom. Talk to these voices as you might speak to disruptive children in a kindergarten class.

4. **Tell yourself (if need be with the help of a counselor) positive, optimistic, hopeful stories.** Stories of hope, faith, and trust that remind you that this is a large universe with seemingly infinite possibilities. Let go of limiting thoughts. Feed the positive wolf, starve the negative wolf.

I often tell the story of the little girl looking out of a window feeling very sad as she watched the men carrying her brother's dead dog to be buried. Then her grandfather walked in to the room, saw what was happening with the little girl, and immediately said, "Oh, Ruth, come over here and look out of this other window. The rose bush you planted is in bloom and looks so beautiful." Then he said "Thee was looking out of the wrong window, dear." This story reminds us to recognize the not-so-cheerful window we may have been looking through, and what we can do about it. We need to simply turn from the window of sadness and feelings of despair and look out of the window of hope, beauty, and all possibilities.

5. **Get rest!** Resting can be very restorative. Often we are so busy we fail to listen to our bodies. Fatigue can bring on or perpetuate negative feelings. It is not uncommon to see some minor task or situation late in the evening as almost impossible to surmount, whereas when one is fresh and well-rested in the morning the same task or situation seems easy to accomplish or address. Therefore, it is important to include rest as part of your program for good mental and physical health.

6. **Follow your creative impulse.** Another aspect for being healthy is to honor your creative impulse. That means if you get the urge to write a poem, paint or draw a picture, do some craft, to bake or cook, or even to write yourself a new positive story to follow, do it. Expressing one's self is important; some psychotherapists have

observed that by suppressing or not honoring in some way (even if it is daydreaming) that creative urge actually may create an imbalance or add to one's depression.

7. **It is important to have a purpose.** Often one relegates purpose to having a job of some kind. Pursuing a goal such as a career certainly gives purpose to one's life. However, there are almost infinite numbers of ways that a person could follow that would give the feeling of purpose. Things such as volunteering, being a friend, helping others, serving your community, and any number of activities could help an individual feel they had a purpose. Many of those serving the very ill and dying have reported that often a person in such extreme circumstances sees what they call, "Their true purpose in life." They say that they have come to realize that their true purpose in life is to love one another, including one's self. This may seem beyond what a person suffering from depression could consider, yet it may be the very key to looking beyond one's personal concerns. Moving beyond the level of the problem and introducing the new element of selflessness, compassion, and love without conditions could be a key element in restoring harmony and balance.

8. **Community, the sense of belonging to a group or community, is important.** Feeling a part of something has been found to be very helpful in restoring harmony and balance to the individual. The need for community can be filled simply by the feeling of belonging to something or someone. This could be a village, an organization, a family, or just having a group of friends with whom you can share and interact. It has been stated by a respected psychiatrist that, "If you don't like the state of your brain you can change it by changing social relationships." There again is the acknowledgement of the importance of community and all the word implies regarding relationships.

9. **Practice some form of meditation and in addition to the meditation practice, think, read, and say to yourself positive affirmations.** Facilitate the feeding of the "good wolf" with positive, affirming statements about yourself, others, and life in general.

Now you have nine specific areas to investigate and to practice in helping to empower you as you proceed on your journey toward harmony and balance.

The person suffering depression has fear. This fear may be acknowledged or go unrecognized; in either case it is important to acknowledge that at some level there is fear.

It has been said that "Fear may be generated by a person fearing they will not get what they want or the fear of losing what they have." By encouraging positive thought patterns through any or all of the above suggestions the grip of attachment will weaken, therefore reducing fearfulness. As the attachment to things being a certain way (the way you think they should be) relaxes, faith and trust become stronger and fear is reduced. As you have more faith and trust in the larger picture and do the best you can at the time, you will find it easier to take things as they come (again reducing fear). You will be able to say to yourself, "Well this is how it is, maybe it is not how I'd planned or ideally would like it to be, but this is the situation and I will work with how it is."

For each step we take to take responsibility for our actions, be they emotional or physical, we gain more control over our behavior. This leads to attitudes that encourage a positive outlook on life and weaken tendencies toward feeling despair, hopelessness, depression. Taking personal responsibility helps replace the victim mentality and is an aid in releasing one from being held hostage by their own mind.

(Used with permission of the author.)

ABOUT THE AUTHOR

Professor John I. Mosher received his PhD from Utah State University in 1972. He taught zoology, field biology, ecology, and mammalogy for the State University of New York for over thirty years. Since retirement he continues to work as a relationship and lifestyles counselor in upstate New York.

CHAPTER 14

CASE HISTORIES

Here are some cases I (BHJ) have worked with. In all of them, the conventional medical drug treatment was either insufficient or resulted in side effects. Most of the patients wanted to try vitamins or other natural treatments. In a couple of cases the psychiatrist suggested an orthomolecular treatment, as all conventional treatment had not been successful. When the new treatment helped, most of these patients were able to either reduce the conventional drugs or put them away.

It is important to note that, in all of these varied cases, successful orthomolecular treatment had the following characteristics:

1. It gave a better effect.

2. It lessened the bad side effects of the conventional drug treatments.

3. It had good side effects.

4. It is economically cheaper.

5. It is environmentally friendly.

 THYROID HORMONE IN TREATMENT-RESISTANT DEPRESSION

Beth had depressions since her teens, two or three times a year, most often in spring and summer. At twenty-eight she was hospitalized when she planned to jump in front of a subway train. According to medical records she may have been psychotic at the time. At forty-one she was in a long depressive episode without psychotic symptoms. Selective serotonin uptake inhibitors (SSRI) did not help. She switched to ven-lafaxin, but got bruises. She got a partial response after changing to nortriptyline (one of the old tricyclic antidepressants), 150 milligrams (mg) daily. Her thyroid blood tests were normal, but she was tired and felt cold. Beth recovered from her depression completely when the thyroid hormone triiodothyronine (T_3), 40 micrograms (mcg) daily, was added, and she was able to go back to her job after a long sick leave. She has since been stable for three years.

 ### CASE 2 — CARBOHYDRATE REDUCTION AND CHROMIUM IN ATYPICAL DEPRESSION; VITAMIN D IN WINTER DEPRESSION

Carla was fifty years old. She had seasonal affective disorder with atypical traits and carbohydrate craving every winter. For twenty years she had used antidepressants during the dark half-year but was troubled by side effects. She wanted to discuss other forms of treatment and was referred for a second opinion. She was advised to avoid sugar and reduce her carbohydrate intake, and to take chromium picolinate 200 mcg three times a day and vitamin D_3 2,000–4,000 International Units (IU) daily. During the following two winters she felt better without using antidepressants.

CASE 3 — NIACIN IN RECURRENT DEPRESSION

Bill was a sixty-seven-year-old man. He mostly had troubles with depressive episodes, but sometimes he also had intermittent explosive aggression and had even hit people close to him a few times. From age twenty-nine to thirty-one he used lithium, which had a stabilizing effect. Then he did not take lithium for six years and had more episodes of depression. From age thirty-seven to sixty-one he took lithium again with good results, but he relapsed when he tried going without it once more.

For years Bill had been treated with lithium, carbamazepine, antidepressants, anxiolytics, and psychotherapy. At the age of sixty he had problems in his job as headmaster in a high-school. He was on lithium, an antidepressant, an anti-anxiety medication, and a sleeping pill. Still, he felt anxious, depressed, and irritated. Then 2,000 mg niacin daily (in an extended release form) was added to Bill's regimen. After three weeks he stopped worrying, and after six weeks he said, "For the first time in ten years I feel I am walking on solid ground instead of a swamp. I was surprised it was such a big difference. Now I have no suicidal thoughts, which I usually have had. I am positive, calmer, sleep better and my blood pressure is normalized." When stressed at his job Bill was able to face his problems in an adequate way. He did not need an anxiolytic pill and he soon stopped using sleep medication. After half a year the antidepressant was stopped, and two months later he also ceased lithium treatment. He felt more alert and sensitive in a positive way, although he was slightly depressed for one month just after he discontinued lithium.

Bill has continued to feel well for the subsequent six years. He forgot to bring the niacin when he travelled a few times, and twice he tested not taking it. Every time he got nervous, irritated, itchy, and restless after two to three days and people around him pointed this out to him. He got better within twelve to twenty-four hours after restarting the niacin, 1000 mg, twice a day.

 ## MICRONUTRIENT TREATMENT FOR RECURRENT DEPRESSION

Gina was seventy-five years old. She had suffered from recurrent depressions during the dark winter season. Light therapy or travelling to lighter and warmer places helped her some winters. She did not want to take any more drugs than she already did for asthma, gout, herpes zoster, hypertension, infections, and muscle rheumatism and her renal function had decreased as well. She was interested in less toxic treatments. Blood testing showed that she had low zinc levels, so she was given zinc supplements. After magnesium supplementation was added she no longer had muscle spasms in one of her feet. With these supplements, together with the B vitamins, vitamin C, and D, she felt more stable, slept better, and had less pain. An important factor in her improvement was her search for better treatments and her positive attitude despite both physical and mental problems.

NIACINAMIDE FOR COMBINED
DEPRESSION AND ANXIETY SYNDROME

Sara was thirty-nine years old and referred from a primary care physician. She had used different antidepressants earlier, but they gave her unacceptable side effects. She had stopped taking an antidepressant drug a month earlier as she wanted to become pregnant. However, she then became more nervous and she asked for other treatment options. She was prescribed three daily capsules of niacinamide, 500 mg, and reported fewer anxiety attacks two weeks later. During the following month she increased her dosage to six capsules a day. For the first two days she was nauseous, but she continued with the 3,000 milligrams a day dosage and found that it decreased anxiety and depressive symptoms. She also recognized that she felt better when she avoided sugar and decreased her carbohydrate intake. At a follow-up two and a half years later she reported that she was taking niacinamide most of the time. She had not used it for six weeks once and felt less stable and more nervous. She was convinced that this treatment made her more calm and fit.

CASE 6   OMEGA-3 FATS FOR DEPRESSION

Lene, fifty-eight years old, had bipolar disorder type II. She was treated with lithium for several years. She started taking 2 grams of omega-3 capsules on her own, as she read it would be good for cardiovascular health. She noticed that her fall seasonal depressions became milder and told her doctor about it. He replied that omega-3 fatty acids may help against depression, but usually not against hypomania. Together with her psychiatrist she was able to reduce her lithium dose, which decreased its side effects.

 ## PHYSICAL ACTIVITY AND BETTER FOOD
FOR DEPRESSION TREATMENT

Harry, fifty-four years old, was a manual worker who previously had never been depressed in his life. However, when he lost his job he became depressed and went to his doctor. Treatment with antidepressant drugs helped only partially, and Harry became overweight, which made him even more depressed. After a year he started to look for a psychiatrist who would be interested in helping him get out of this vicious circle. He was disappointed with the meager help available from prescription medicines and realized he needed to make some changes himself. Harry reviewed his lifestyle with his psychiatrist's support, and decided to change his eating habits. Harry had always been a meat eater. Now he changed some of his meat to fish, stopped eating bread, and reduced his carbohydrate intake. He also started to go bicycling every day and felt more vigorous. Within six months he was able to stop taking antidepressants and he got a job as a professional bus driver.

CASE 8 MICRONUTRIENT TREATMENT IN BIPOLAR DISORDER TYPE II

Karen was sixty-four years old. She told her psychiatrist she had stopped taking lithium and thyroid medication after seeing a natural therapist. Instead Karen was taking vitamin and mineral supplements. Some herbal preparations, which the doctor did not know anything about, had been recommended for her thyroid. A consultation with her psychiatrist was arranged after a nervous phone call from one of her two daughters. The doctor explained that taking away important medication such as lithium right away could be dangerous, given her bipolar disorder type II. The patient was very persistent that she would not go back on the medication, but agreed to bring her daughters for the following week's visit. The patient was more nervous and her mood less stable on this visit with her daughters. Then a plan was worked out so Karen visited the doctor more frequently and increased the dosages of the supplements that might help stabilize mood. This required that she took magnesium, zinc, vitamins B, C, D, and omega-3 in adequate doses. She got much better the following two months and felt less subdued than before. Her thyroid blood test results were acceptable. During the following year she got more stable with a combination of thyroid hormones T_4 and T_3, and she did not need to reintroduce lithium into her program.

AT THE CROSSROADS FOR ALL THE DIFFERENCE

Two roads diverged in a wood, and I—
I took the one less travelled by,
And that has made all the difference.
—ROBERT FROST (1874–1963)

Wherever you are, there are different roads to take. Some of them are difficult to find; their entrance may be blocked by bushes and shadows. When you recognize the entrance, it is still unknown what you will find further down the road. Sometimes you go in one direction only to realize it is better to turn around and head for another path. It is easy to see the flashy neon sign pointing to Route T (toximolecular), accompanied by the "travel my way, this is the highway that is best" messages shouting from the loud-speakers. Most of us are familiar with what is sold along this way. This is where you get the compounds that are foreign to the body, expensive, and highly promoted. Sometimes these remedies help, at least for a time. When they do not work or, even worse, hurt you, this is denied or explained away. Besides being expensive, it is clear that many of these pharmaceutical drugs are toxic to humans and the ecosphere.

You may have noticed that the entrance ramp onto the interstate highway often gets jammed because of troubles further down the road. Reflecting on this, you may find there are many other directions available to examine in your personal terrain. Lesser known is Route O (orthomolecular). Most people do not see it at first, especially if they

177

are not looking for it and have been diverted by the highly promoted road. It is an older road. What is offered here are the natural substances familiar to the body over millions of years. These solutions are usually safer, cheaper, and often comparatively effective. You may have to walk along to review these options, and consider other roads as well to find what you want and what works for you. It is important that you always think for yourself.

FINDING RELIABLE INFORMATION ON ORTHOMOLECULAR MEDICINE

*"Freedom of the press is guaranteed only
to those who own one."*
—ABBOTT JOSEPH LIEBLING (1904–1963)

NEGATIVE BIAS ON THE INTERNET

Hundreds of millions of people search the Internet daily for health information, but what exactly are they getting? A November, 2012 Google search on the keyword "health" retrieved over 4 billion results. Still, information about orthomolecular medicine is entirely absent at many of the largest and most frequented "health" websites. Therefore, when the layman searches for nutritional therapy, they often get false or misleading information from a pharmaphilic (drug-loving) viewpoint. Pharmaceutical medicine's influence on the Internet is very strong, although less dominant than its enormous presence on television and in print media.

On the medical Internet, "reliable" or "carefully selected" seem to mean selection that purposefully excludes orthomolecular medicine. Is there a medical blacklist, and if so, is orthomolecular medicine on it? Terms such as "reliable" and "carefully selected" are meant to imply some kind of objective editing, but when the entire discipline of orthomolecular medicine is excluded, it is in fact censorship by selection.

NEGATIVE BIAS IN GOVERNMENT

The world's largest medical library is biased. The United States National Library of Medicine indexes thousands of medical journals and makes them instantly accessible through their electronic MEDLINE (Medical Literature Analysis and Retrieval System Online) database. NLM and MEDLINE are operated at taxpayer expense.

The peer-reviewed *Journal of Orthomolecular Medicine* (*JOM*), continually published for over forty years, remains conspicuous by its absence from the library's listings. *JOM* publishes high-dose vitamin therapy studies and is read by physicians and scientists in over thirty-five countries. There were 754 million MEDLINE searches in the year 2005, and not one of those searches found a single article from *JOM*. Since then, there have been literally billions of searches on MEDLINE, and not one of *those* ever found a *JOM* paper, either. Odd, really, since the *Journal of Orthomolecular Medicine* has been published for four decades. It has an editorial review board of physicians and university researchers. And, *JOM* has published papers by prominent scientists, including two-time Nobel Prize winner Linus Pauling, Ph.D. Critics accuse NLM of information censorship, which, they maintain, is grossly inappropriate for a public library.

And MEDLINE, to this day (March 2012) still steadfastly refuses to index the *Journal of Orthomolecular Medicine*.

By excluding the *Journal of Orthomolecular Medicine* and certain other journals from its MEDLINE/PubMed indexing services, the U.S. National Library of Medicine (NLM) has limited doctors' access to information. At one time, limits were understandable; only 239 journals were indexed when MEDLINE first went online in 1971. MEDLINE became freely available on the Internet in June of 1997, and now, fifteen years later, indexes over 5,000 journals. Interestingly, it is the Internet itself that has made MEDLINE obsolete. The 'net offers numerous search engines and indexing services for professionals and public alike.

Uncensored Science

Search engines such as Google Scholar (http://scholar.google.com) are now a primary resource for scientists and academics. Google Scholar indexes MEDLINE itself, but this constitutes only a fraction of its information base. Google Scholar also shows web pages for a journal, the authors, and frequently an independent PDF copy of an article itself. Furthermore, Google Scholar allows libraries and publishers to index their collections, including abstracts and direct links to obtain the complete article. Google Scholar also indexes government sites, university lecture notes, academic presentations, scientific conferences, and, potentially, any relevant material available or linked to the Internet.

Medical information access has reached a tipping point. It is no longer possible for agencies such as NLM to obstruct rapid access to journals it chooses to exclude. Those who want information can find it just as fast via Google Scholar as they can with MEDLINE, and Google Scholar is far more comprehensive. Google Scholar indexes the *Journal of Orthomolecular Medicine*. Indeed, any Internet search engine can find the entire online *JOM* archives at http://orthomolecular.org/library/jom.

But not by using taxpayer-funded MEDLINE. To be fair, it must be admitted that in May 2007, NLM acknowledged that it does physically have *JOM* on its shelves, saying in correspondence: "While we hold the *Journal of Orthomolecular Medicine* in our print collection here at NLM, it is not currently indexed for MEDLINE/PubMed."

One might well wonder why NLM, a taxpayer-supported public library, physically archives a journal, and yet refuses to index it. Dr. Harold D. Foster has wryly observed that "MEDLINE treats the *Journal* like a dirty magazine: to be read privately, but the fact kept hidden from the public."

MEDLINE limits access to scientific data by exercising control over which journals it includes. Oddly enough, *Time, Newsweek, Consumer Reports,* and even *Reader's Digest* are included in MEDLINE. Conversely, important publications that show maverick tendencies, such as the journal *Fluoride,* the *Journal of American Physicians and Surgeons, Medical Veritas,* and the *Journal of Nutritional and Ecological Medicine* are excluded from MEDLINE. The idea that the *Reader's Digest* is of greater clinical utility than these journals is clearly absurd.

But Abraham Lincoln was right: you cannot fool all of the people all of the time.

MEDLINE Obsolescence

When it began in 1971, MEDLINE was the only game in town. We are now witnessing the end of MEDLINE's era as the premiere source of medical information. While it remains heavily used, it is fast losing its dominance to Google Scholar. Given time, additional indexing services will enhance the delivery of information to doctors, scientists, and medical professionals.

The U.S. National Library of Medicine appears to have forgotten that human beings are historically intolerant of censorship, and have rarely responded positively to it. "In the long run of history," wrote Alfred Whitney Griswold, "the censor and the inquisitor have always lost."

We are now entering a new era of medical informatics. The wide availability of information on the safety and effectiveness of nutritional therapies is changing healthcare. People have tried orthomolecular medicine for themselves and found it effective. Before too long, the wisdom of patients, backed by the pressure of hundreds of millions of Internet searches, may drag conventional doctors, kicking and screaming, into the orthomolecular information age.

It will be a birth worth attending.

RECOMMENDED
READING

You know what is really depressing? The number of books on depression that do not even mention the word "niacin." It's true; try a search and see. Over a dozen of the best-selling "get rid of depression" books do not have a single comment on the most important therapies of all: vitamin B_3, niacin. Fortunately, there are a quite a few that emphasize nutrition, and we want you to read as much as possible.

Our recommendations for good books to start with include:

Atkins, R. C. *Dr. Atkins' Vita-Nutrient Solution: Nature's Answer to Drugs.* New York: Simon & Schuster, 1998.

Barsky, A. J., E. C. Deans. *Feeling Better: The 6-Week Mind-Body Program to Ease Your Chronic Symptoms.* New York: Collins, 2006.

Baumel, S. *Dealing with Depression Naturally: Complementary and Alternative Therapies for Restoring Emotional Health.* 2nd ed. Los Angeles: Keats Pub., 2000.

Birkmayer, G. D. *NADH: The Biological Hydrogen: The Secret of Our Life Energy.* Laguna Beach, CA: Basic Health, 2009.

Challem, J. *The Food-Mood Solution: All-Natural Ways to Banish Anxiety, Depression, Anger, Stress, Overeating, and Alcohol and Drug Problems—and Feel Good Again.* Hoboken, NJ: John Wiley & Sons, 2008.

Cheraskin, E., W. M. Ringsdorf, A. Brecher. *Psychodietetics: Food as the Key to Emotional Health.* New York: Bantam Books, 1974.

Edelman, E. *Natural Healing for Bipolar Disorder: A Compendium of Nutritional Approaches.* Borage Books, 2009.

Gaby, A. R. *Nutritional Medicine.* Fritz Perlberg Publishing, 2011.

Greenblatt, J. *The Breakthrough Depression Solution.* North Branch, MN: Sunrise River Press, 2011.

Growden, A. "Neurotransmitter Precursors in the Diet," in *Nutrition and the Brain,* R. J. Wurtman, J. J. Wurtman., Eds., 117–181, Raven Press, 1979.

Guyol, G. *Who's Crazy Here?* Stonington, CT: Ajoite Publishing, 2010.

Hawkins, D., L. Pauling. *Orthomolecular Psychiatry: Treatment of Schizophrenia.* San Francisco: W. H. Freeman, 1973

Hedaya, R. J. *The Antidepressant Survival Guide: The Clinically Proven Program to Enhance the Benefits and Beat the Side Effects of Your Medication.* New York: Three Rivers, 2000.

Hickey, S., A. W. Saul. *Vitamin C: The Real Story.* Laguna Beach, CA: Basic Health, 2008.

Hickey, S., H. Roberts. *Tarnished Gold: The Sickness of Evidence-Based Medicine.* CreateSpace, 2011.

Hoffer, A., A. W. Saul. *Orthomolecular Medicine for Everyone: Megavitamin Therapeutics for Families and Physicians.* Laguna Beach, CA: Basic Health, 2008.

Hoffer, A., A. W. Saul. *The Vitamin Cure for Alcoholism: How to Protect Against and Fight Alcoholism Using Nutrition and Vitamin Supplementation.* Laguna Beach, CA: Basic Health, 2009.

Hoffer, A., A. W. Saul, H. D. Foster. *Niacin: The Real Story.* Laguna Beach, CA: Basic Health, 2012.

Hoffer A., H. D. Foster. *Feel Better, Live Longer with Vitamin B_3: Nutrient Deficiency and Dependency.* Toronto, ONT: CCNM Press, 2007.

Hoffer, A., M. Walker, M. *Orthomolecular Nutrition: New Lifestyle for Super Good Health.* New Canaan, CT: Keats, 1978.

Huemer, R. P. "Brain Food: Neurotransmitters Make You Think," *Let's Live,* December, 1981.

Iliardi, S. S. *The Depression Cure: The 6-Step Program to Beat Depression Without Drugs.* Cambridge, MA: Da Capo Lifelong, 2009.

Knittel, L. *User's Guide to Natural Remedies for Depression: Learn about Safe and Natural Treatments to Uplift Your Mood and Conquer Depression.* North Bergen, NJ: Basic Health, 2003.

Kohlstadt, I. (editor). *Food and Nutrients in Disease Management.* CRC Press, 2009.

Larson, J. M. *Depression-Free, Naturally: 7 Weeks to Eliminating Anxiety, Despair, Fatigue, and Anger from Your Life.* New York: Wellspring/Ballantine, 2001.

Lilliston, L. *Megavitamins: A New Key to Health.* Greenwich, CT: Fawcett Publications, 1975.

McCracken, R. D. *Niacin and Human Health Disorders.* Hygea, 1994.

McLeod, M. N. *Lifting Your Depression: How a Psychiatrist Discovered Chromium's Role in the Treatment of Depression,* 2nd ed. Laguna Beach, CA: Basic Health, 2009.

Murray, M. T. *5-HTP: The Natural Way to Overcome Depression, Obesity, and Insomnia.* New York: Bantam Books, 1998.

Nutrition News, Vol. 2, No. 9, 1979

Passwater, R. *Supernutrition.,* New York: Pocket Books, 1975.

Pauling, L. *How To Live Longer and Feel Better.* 20th anniversary edition. Corvallis, OR: Oregon State University Press, 2006.

Pfeiffer, C. C. *Nutrition and Mental Illness: An Orthomolecular Approach to Balancing Body Chemistry.* Rochester, VT: Healing Arts Press, 1988.

Ravnskov, U. *Ignore the Awkward! How the Cholesterol Myths Are Kept Alive.* CreateSpace, 2010.

Rose, A., A. Adams. *Rebuild from Depression: A Nutrient Guide Including Depression in Pregnancy and Postpartum.* California Hot Springs, CA: Purple Oak Press, 2009.

Schachter, M. B., D. Mitchell. *What Your Doctor May Not Tell You About Depression: The Breakthrough All-Natural Solution for Effective Treatment.* New York: Warner Wellness, 2006.

Shames R. L., K. H. Shames. *Thyroid Power: 10 Steps to Total Health.* New York: Harper Collins, 2001.

Walsh, W. J. *Nutrient Power: Heal Your Biochemistry and Heal Your Brain.* New York: Skyhorse Publishing, 2012.

Werbach, M. *Nutritional Influences on Mental Illness.* 2nd ed. Tarzana, CA: Third Line Press, 1999.

Whitaker, R. *Anatomy of an Epidemic: Magic Bullets, Psychiatric Drugs, and the Astonishing Rise of Mental Illness in America.* New York: Crown, 2010.

Before you buy a book on rock music, make sure it at least *mentions* the guitar. Before you buy a book on Shakespeare, make sure it at least *mentions Hamlet.* A book on depression without niacin is like, well, a lot like having depression and not taking niacin.

If you have not tried niacin and the other measures we have discussed in this book, now is your chance. If this seems too cheap and too simple, you are certainly free to make it all as complicated as your psychoanalyst budget and prescription drug plan will allow.

REFERENCES

Chapter 1: The Plague of Depression

1. Murray, C. J. L., A. D. Lopez. "Evidence-Based Health Policy—Lessons from the Global Burden of Disease Study." *Science* 274(5288) (Nov 1, 1996):740–743.

2. Costello, E. J., D. S. Pine, C. Hammen, et al. "Development and Natural History of Mood Disorders." *Biol Psychiatry* 52(6) (Sep 2002):529–542.

3. Hagnell, O., J. Lanke, B. Rorsman, et al. "Are We Entering an Age of Melancholy? Depressive Illness in a Prospective Epidemiological Study over 25 Years: The Lundby Study, Sweden." *Psychol Med* 12(2) (May 1982):279–289.

4. Rutter, M., D. J. Smith. *Psychosocial Disorders in Young People: Time Trends and Their Causes.* Chichester: John Wiley & Sons, 1995.

5. Murphy, H. B., B. M. Taumoepeau. "Traditionalism and Mental Health in the South Pacific: A Re-Examination of an Old Hypothesis." *Psychol Med* 10(3) (Aug 1980):471–482. Brody, H. *The Other Side of Eden: Hunters, Farmers, and the Shaping of the World.* New York: North Point Press, 2001. McGrath-Hanna, N. K., D. M. Greene, R. J. Tavernier, et al. "Diet and Mental Health in the Arctic: Is Diet an Important Factor for Mental Health in Circumpolar Peoples?—A Review." *Int J Circumpolar Health* 62(3) (Sep 2003):228–241.

6. Frances, A. "Whither DSM-V?" *Br J Psychiatry* 195(5) (Nov 2009):391–392. Frances, A. "The First Draft of DSM-V." *BMJ* 340(7745) (Mar 2010):492.

7. Horwitz, A. V., J. C. Wakefield. *The Loss of Sadness: How Psychiatry Transformed Normal Sorrow into Depressive Disorder.* New York: Oxford University Press, 2007.

8. Frances, A., H. L. Egger. "Whither Psychiatric Diagnosis." *Aust N Z J Psychiatry* 33(2) (Apr 1999):161–165.

9. Van Praag, H. M. "No Functional Psychopharmacology without Functional Psychopathology." *Acta Psychiatr Scand* 122(6) (Dec 2010):438–439.

10. Winokur, G. "All Roads Lead to Depression: Clinically Homogeneous, Etiologically Heterogeneous." *J Affect Disord* 45(1–2) (Aug 1997):97–108.

11. Chisholm, D., P. Diehr, M. Knapp, et al. "Depression Status, Medical Comorbidity and Resource Costs. Evidence from an International Study of Major Depression in Primary Care (LIDO)." *Br J Psychiatry* 183(2) (Aug 2003):121–131.

12. Horrobin, D. F., C. N. Bennett. "Depression and Bipolar Disorder: Relationships to Impaired Fatty Acid and Phospholipid Metabolism and to Diabetes, Cardiovascular Disease, Immunological Abnormalities, Cancer, Ageing and Osteoporosis. Possible Candidate Genes." *Prostaglandins Leukot Essent Fatty Acids* 60(:4) (1999):217–234.

13. Björntorp, P. "Visceral Obesity: A "Civilization Syndrome." *Obes Res* 1(3) (May 1993):206–222.

14. Stewart, T. D., S. A. Atlas. "Syndrome X, Depression, and Chaos: Relevance to Medical Practice." *Conn Med* 64(6) (Jun 2000):343–345.

15. Newman, J. C., R. J. Holden. "The 'Cerebral Diabetes' Paradigm for Unipolar Depression." *Med Hypotheses* 41(5) (Nov 1993):391–408.

16. McIntyre, R. S., J. K. Soczynska, J. Z. Konarski, et al. "Should Depressive Syndromes Be Reclassified as "Metabolic Syndrome Type II"?" *Ann Clin Psychiatry* 19(4) (Oct-Dec 2007):257–264.

17. Harvey, B. H. "Is Major Depressive Disorder a Metabolic Encephalopathy?" *Hum Psychopharmacol* 23(5) (Jul 2008):371–384.

18. McIntyre, R. S., N. L. Rasgon, D. E. Kemp, et al. "Metabolic Syndrome and Major Depressive Disorder: Co-Occurence and Pathophysiologic Overlap." *Curr Diab Rep* 9(1) (Feb 2009):51–59. Zeugmann, S., A. Quante, I. Heuser, et al. "Inflammatory Biomarkers in 70 Depressed Inpatients with and without the Metabolic Syndrome." *J Clin Psychiatry* 71(8) (Aug 2010):1007–1016.

19. Csikszentmihalyi, M. "If We Are So Rich, Why Aren't We Happy?" *Am Psychol* 54(10) (Oct 1999):821–827. Lane, R. E. *The Loss of Happiness in Market Democracies.* New Haven, CT: Yale University Press, 2000.

20. Kendler, K. S., J. M. Hettema, F. Butera, et al. "Life Event Dimensions of Loss, Humiliation, Entrapment, and Danger in the Prediction of Onsets of Major Depression and Generalized Anxiety." *Arch Gen Psychiatry* 60(8) (Aug 2003):789–796.

21. Capuron, L., S. Schroecksnadel, C. Féart, et al. "Chronic Low-Grade Inflammation in Elderly Persons Is Associated with Altered Tryptophan and Tyrosine Metabolism: Role in Neuropsychiatric Symptoms." *Biol Psychiatry* 70(2) (Jul 15, 2011):175–82.

22. Charlton, B. "The Malaise Theory of Depression: Major Depressive Disorder is Sickness Behavior and Antidepressants Are Analgesics." *Med Hypotheses* 54(1) (Jan 2000):126–130.

23. Pauling, L. "Orthomolecular Psychiatry. Varying the Concentrations of Substances Normally Present in the Human Body May Control Mental Disease." *Science* 160(3825) (Apr 19, 1968):265–271.

24. Mayer, A. M. "Historical Changes in the Mineral Content of Fruits and Vegetables." *Br Food J* 99(6) (1997):207–211. Davis, D. R., M. D. Epp, H. D. Riordan. "Changes in USDA Food Composition Data for 43 Garden Crops, 1950 to 1999." *J Am Coll Nutr* 23(6) (Dec 2004):669–682. Thomas, D. "The Mineral Depletion of Foods Available to Us as a Nation (1940–2002)—A Review of the 6th Edition of McCance and Widdowson." *Nutr Health* 19(1–2) (2007):21–55. Ekholm, P., H. Reinivuo, P. Mattila. "Changes in the Mineral and Trace Element Contents of Cereals, Fruits and Vegetables in Finland." *J Food Comp Anal* 20(6) (2007):487–495.

25. Cordain, L., B. A. Watkins, G. L. Florant. "Fatty Acid Analysis of Wild Ruminant Tissues: Evolutionary Implications for Reducing Diet-Related Chronic Disease." *Eur J Clin Nutr* 56(3) (Mar 2002):181–191.

26. Louv, R. *Last Child in the Woods: Saving Our Children from Nature-Deficit Disorder.* Chapel Hill, NC: Algonquin Books, 2008.

27. Louv, R. *The Nature Principle: Human Restoration and the End of Nature-Deficit Disorder.* Chapel Hill, NC: Algonquin Books, 2011.

28. Healy, D. *The Antidepressant Era.* Cambridge, MA: Harvard University Press, 1997.

29. Shepherd, M. "The Placebo: From Specificity to the Non-Specific and Back." *Psychol Med* 23(3) (Aug 1993):569–578. Walsh, B. T., S. N. Seidman, R. Sysko, et al. "Placebo Response in Studies of Major Depression: Variable, Substantial, and Growing." *JAMA* 287(14) (Apr 10, 2002):1840–1847.

30. Kirsch, I., B. J. Deacon, T. B. Huedo-Medina, et al. "Initial Severity and Antidepressant Benefits: A Meta-Analysis of Data Submitted to the Food and Drug Administration." *PLoS Med* 5(2) (Feb 2008): e45. Fournier, J. C., R. J. DeRubeis, S. D. Hollon, et al. "Antidepressant Drug Effects and Depression Severity: A Patient-Level Meta-Analysis." *JAMA* 303(1) (Jan 6, 2010):47–53.

31. Insel, T. R., P. S. Wang. "The STAR*D Trial: Revealing the Need for Better Treatments." *Psychiatr Serv* 60(11) (Nov 2009):1466–1467.

32. Fava, G. A., E. Offidani. "The Mechanisms of Tolerance in Antidepressant Action." *Prog Neuropsychopharmacol Biol Psychiatry* 35(7) (Aug 15, 2011):1593–1602. Whitaker, R. *Anatomy of an Epidemic: Magic Bullets, Psychiatric Drugs, and the Astonishing Rise of Mental Illness in America.* New York: Crown, 2010.

33. Cuijpers, P. "Examining the Effects of Preventive Programs on the Incidence of New Cases of Mental Disorders: The Lack of Statistical Power." *Am J Psychiatry* 160(8) (Aug 2003):1385–1391. Jané-Llopis, E., C. Hosman, R. Jenkins, et al. "Predictors of Efficacy in Depression Programmes: Meta-Analysis." *Br J Psychiatry* 183(5) (Nov 2003):384–397. Bramesfeld, A., M. Wismar. "Mental Health Promotion and Prevention of Mental Health Disorders: Highly Needed But Realistic?" *Eurohealth* 9 (2003):34–35.

Chapter 2: An Evolutionary View of Depression

1. Therborn, G. *The World: A Beginner's Guide.* Cambridge, UK: Polity, 2011.

2. Engel, G. L. "The Need for a New Medical Model: A Challenge for Biomedicine." *Science* 196(4286) (Apr 1977):129–136. Engel, G. L. "The Clinical Application of the Biopsychosocial Model." *Am J Psychiatry* 137(5) (May 1980):535–544. Engel, G. L. "How Much Longer Must Medicine's Science Be Bound by a Seventeenth Century World View?" *Psychother Psychosom* 57(1–2) (1992):3–16.

3. Kitano, H. "Systems Biology: A Brief Overview." *Science* 295(5560) (Mar 1, 2002):1662–1664.

4. Nesse, R. M., G. C. Williams. *Why We Get Sick: The New Science of Darwinian Medicine.* New York: Vintage Books, 1994.

5. McGuire, M. T., A. Troisi. *Darwinian Psychiatry.* New York: Oxford University

Press, 1998. Stevens, A., J. Price. *Evolutionary Psychiatry: A New Beginning.* 2nd Edition. London: Routledge, 2000.

6. Nesse, R. M. "Is Depression an Adaptation?" *Arch Gen Psychiatry* 57(1) (Jan 2000):14–20. Rohde, P. "The Relevance of Hierarchies, Territories, Defeat for Depression in Humans: Hypotheses and Clinical Predictions." *J Affect Disord* 65(3) (Aug 2001):221–30.

7. Eaton, S. B., M. Shostak, M. Konner. *The Paleolithic Prescription: A Program of Diet and Exercise and a Design for Living.* New York: Harper & Row, 1988.

8. Stevens, A., J. Price. *Evolutionary Psychiatry: A New Beginning.* 2nd Edition. London: Routledge, 2000.

9. O'Keefe, J. H., L. Cordain. "Cardiovascular Disease Resulting from a Diet and Lifestyle at Odds with Our Paleolithic Genome: How to Become a 21st-Century Hunter-Gatherer." *Mayo Clin Proc* 79(1) (Jan 2004):101–108.

10. Sharma, A. M. "The Thrifty-Genotype Hypothesis and Its Implications for the Study of Complex Genetic Disorders in Man." *J Mol Med* 76(8) (Jul 1998):568–571.

11. Poston, W. S. 2nd, J. P. Foreyt. "Obesity Is an Environmental Issue." *Atherosclerosis* 146(2) (Oct 1999):201–209.

12. Caspi, A., K. Sugden, T. E. Moffit, et al. "Influence of Life Stress on Depression: Moderation by a Polymorphism of the 5-HTT Gene." *Science* 301(5631) (Jul 18, 2003):386–389. Keers, R., R. Uher. "Gene-Environment Interaction in Major Depression and Antidepressant Treatment Response." *Curr Psychiatry Rep* 14(2) (Apr 2012):129–137.

13. Post, R. M. "Preface and Overview." *Clin Neurosci Res* 2(3–4) (2002):122–126.

14. Willet, W. "Balancing Life-Style and Genomics Research for Disease Prevention." *Science* 296(5568) (Apr 26, 2002):695–698.

15. Stringer, C. "Human Evolution: Out of Ethiopia." *Nature* 423(6941) (Jun 12, 2003):692–3, 695.

16. Torrey, E. F., J. Miller. *The Invisible Plague: The Rise of Mental Illness from 1750 to the Present.* New Brunswick: Rutgers University Press, 2001.

17. McKibben, B. *The End of Nature.* New York: Random House, 1989.

18. Wilson, E. O. *The Future of Life.* New York: Alfred A Knopf, 2002.

19. Levitt, A. J., M. H. Boyle. "The Impact of Latitude on the Prevalence of Seasonal Depression." *Can J Psychiatry* 47(4) (May 2002):361–367.

20. Karatsoreos, I.N., S. Bhagat, E. B. Bloss, et al. "Disruption of Circadian Clocks has Ramifications for Metabolism, Brain, and Behavior." *Proc Natl Acad Sci U S A* 108(4) (2011):1657–1662.

21. Spiegel, K., R. Leproult, E. Van Cauter. "Impact of Sleep Debt on Metabolic and Endocrine Function." *Lancet* 354(9188) (Oct 23, 1999):1435–1439. Spiegel, K., E. Tasali, R. Leproult, et al. "Effects of Poor and Short Sleep on Glucose Metabolism and Obesity Risk." *Nat Rev Endocrinol* 5(5) (May 2009):253–261.

22. Wiley, T. S., B. Formby. *Lights Out: Sleep, Sugar, and Survival.* New York: Simon & Schuster, 2000.

23. Frumkin, H. "Beyond Toxicity: Human Health and the Natural Environment." *Am J Prev Med* 20(3) (Apr 2001):234–240. Berman, M. G., E. Kross, K. M. Krpan, et al. "Interacting with Nature Improves Cognition and Affect for Individuals with Depression." *J Affect Disord* 140(3) (Mar 31, 2012):300–305.

24. Terman, M., J. S. Terman. "Treatment of Seasonal Affective Disorder with a High-Output Negative Ionizer." *J Altern Complement Med* 1(1) (Jan 1995):87–92.

25. Terman, M., J. S. Terman, D. C. Ross. "A Controlled Trial of Timed Bright Light and Negative Air Ionization for Treatment of Winter Depression." *Arch Gen Psychiatry* 55(10) (Oct 1998):875–882.

26. Küller, R. "The Influence of Light on Circarhythms in Humans." *J Physiol Anthropol Appl Human Sci* 21(2) (Mar 2002):87–91.

27. Wirz-Justice, A., P. Graw, K. Kräuchi, et al. "'Natural' Light Treatment of Seasonal Affective Disorder." *J Affect Disord* 37(2–3) (Apr 12, 1996):109–120.

28. Brown, M. A., J. Goldstein-Shirley, J. Robinson, et al. "The Effects of a Multi-Modal Intervention Trial of Light, Exercise, and Vitamins on Women's Mood." *Women Health* 34(3) (2001):93–112.

29. Cannon, G. "Nutrition: The New World Disorder." *Asia Pacific J Clin Nutr* 11(Suppl. 3) (2002):S498–509.

30. Zimmet, P. "Globalization, Coca-Colonization and the Chronic Disease Epidemic: Can the Doomsday Scenario Be Averted?" *J Intern Med* 247(3) (Mar 2000):301–310. Zimmet, P., C. R. Thomas. "Genotype, Obesity and Cardiovascular Disease—Has Technical and Social Advancement Outstripped Evolution?" *J Intern Med* 254(2) (Aug 2003):114–125.

31. Peet, M. "International Variations in the Outcome of Schizophrenia and the Prevalence of Depression in Relation to National Dietary Practices: An Ecological Analysis." *Br J Psychiatry* 184(5) (May 2004):404–408.

32. Horrobin, D. "Why Do We Not Make More Medical Use of Nutritional Knowledge? How an Inadvertent Alliance between Reductionist Scientists, Holistic Dietitians and Drug-Oriented Regulators and Governments Has Blocked Progress." *Br J Nutr* 90(1) (Jul 2003):233–238.

33. Johannessen, B., I. Skagestad, A. M. Bergkaasa. "Food as Medicine in Psychiatric Care: Which Profession Should Be Responsible for Imparting Knowledge and Use of Omega-3 Fatty Acids in Psychiatry." *Complement Ther Clin Pract* 17(2) (May 2011): 107–112.

34. Marteinsdottir, I., D. F. Horrobin, C. Stenfors, et al. "Changes in Dietary Fatty Acids Alter Phospholipid Fatty Acid Composition in Selected Regions of Rat Brain." *Prog Neuropsychopharmacol Biol Psychiatry* 22(6) (Aug 1998):1007–1021.

35. Puri, B. K., J. Holmes, G. Hamilton. "Eicosapentaenoic Acid-Rich Essential Fatty Acid Supplementation in Chronic Fatigue Syndrome Associated with Symptom Remission and Structural Brain Changes." *Int J Clin Pract* 58(3) (Mar 2004):297–299.

36. Chalon, S., S. Delion-Vancassel, C. Belzung, et al. "Dietary Fish Oil Affects Monoaminergic Neurotransmission and Behavior in Rats." *J Nutr* 128(12) (Dec 1998):2512–2519.

37. Hibbeln, J. "Fish Consumption and Major Depression." *Lancet* 351(9110) (Apr 18, 1998):1213.

38. Nemets, B., Z. Stahl, R. H. Belmaker. "Addition of Omega-3 Fatty Acid to Maintenance Medication Treatment for Recurrent Unipolar Depressive Disorder." *Am J Psychiatry* 159(3) (Mar 2002):477–479. Peet, M., D. F. Horrobin. "A Dose-Ranging Study of the Effects of Ethyl-Eicosapentaenoate in Patients with Ongoing Depression Despite Apparently Adequate Treatment with Standard Drugs." *Arch Gen Psychiatry* 59(10) (Oct 2002):913–919.

39. Su, K. P., S. Y. Huang, C. C. Chiu, et al. "Omega-3 Fatty Acids in Major Depressive Disorder. A Preliminary Double-Blind, Placebo-Controlled Trial." *Eur Neuropsychopharmacol* 13(4) (Aug 2003):267–271.

40. Marangell, L. B., J. M. Martinez, H. A. Zboyan, et al. "A Double-Blind, Placebo-Controlled Study of the Omega-3 Fatty Acid Docosahexaenoic Acid in the Treatment of Major Depression." *Am J Psychiatry* 160(5) (May 2003):996–998.

41. Colantuoni, C., P. Rada, J. McCarthy, et al. "Evidence that Intermittent, Excessive Sugar Intake Causes Endogenous Opioid Dependence." *Obes Res* 10(6) (Jun 2002):478–488.

42. Westover, A. N., L. B. Marangell. "A Cross-National Relationship between Sugar Consumption and Major Depression?" *Depress Anxiety* 16(3) (2002):118–120.

43. Christensen, L., R. Burrows. "Dietary Treatment of Depression." *Behav Ther* 21(2) (Spring 1990):183–193.

44. Cleave, T. L. *The Saccharine Disease: The Master Disease of Our Time.* New Canaan, CT: Keats Publishing, 1975. Dufty, W. *Sugar Blues.* New York: Warner Books, 1975.

45. Harrison, R.A., D. Holt, D. J. Pattison, et al. "Are Those in Need Taking Dietary Supplements? A Survey of 21 923 Adults." *Br J Nutr* 91(4) (Apr 2004):617–623.

46. Alaimo, K., C. M. Olson, E. A. Frongillo. "Family Food Insufficiency, but Not Low Family Income, Is Positively Associated with Dysthymia and Suicide Symptoms in Adolescents." *J Nutr* 132(4) (2002):719–725.

47. Coppen, A., Bailey, J. "Enhancement of the Antidepressant Action of Fluoxetine by Folic Acid: A Randomized, Placebo Controlled Trial." *J Affect Dis* 60(2) (Nov 2000):121–130.

48. Brody, S. "High-Dose Ascorbic Acid Increases Intercourse Frequency and Improves Mood: A Randomized Controlled Clinical Trial." *Biol Psychiatry* 52(4) (Aug 2002):371–374.

49. Lansdowne, A. T., S. C. Provost. "Vitamin D_3 Enhances Mood in Healthy Subjects During Winter." *Psychopharmacology (Berl)* 135(4) (Feb 1998):319–323.

50. Benton, D. "Selenium Intake, Mood and Other Aspects of Physiological Functioning." *Nutr Neurosci* 5(6) (Dec 2002):363–374.

51. Murck, H. "Magnesium and Affective Disorders." *Nutr Neurosci* 5(6) (Dec 2002):375–389.

52. Nowak, G., M. Siwek, D. Dudek, et al. "Effect of Zinc Supplementation on Antidepressant Therapy in Unipolar Depression: A Preliminary Placebo-Controlled Study." *Pol J Pharmacol* 55(6) (Nov-Dec 2003):1143–1147.

53. Davidson, J. R. T., K. Abraham, K. M. Connor, et al. "Effectiveness of Chromium in Atypical Depression: A Placebo-Controlled Trial." *Biol Psychiatry* 53(3) (Feb 1, 2003):261–264.

54. Kobilo, T., Q.-R. Liu, K. Gandhi, et al. "Running is the Neurogenic and Neurotrophic Stimulus in Environmental Enrichment." *Learn Mem* 18(9) (2011):605–609.

55. Cordain, L., R. W. Gotshall, S. B. Eaton, et al. "Physical Activity, Energy Expenditure and Fitness: An Evolutionary Perspective." *Int J Sports Med* 19(5) (Jul 1998):328–335. Booth, F. W., M. V. Chakravarthy, E. Spangenburg. "Exercise and Gene Expression: Physiological Regulation of the Human Genome through Physical Activity." *J Physiol* 543(Pt 2) (Sep 1, 2002):399–411.

56. Jacka, F. N., J. A. Pasco, L. J. Williams, et al. "Lower Levels of Physical Activity in Childhood Associated with Adult Depression." *J Sci Med Sport* 14(3) (May 14, 2011):222–226. Johnson, K. E., L. A. Taliaferro, "Relationships between Physical Activity and Depressive Symptoms among Middle and Older Adolescents: A Review of the Research Literature." *J Spec Pediatr Nurs* 16(4) (2011):235–251.

57. Camacho, T. C., R. E. Roberts, N. B. Lazarus, et al. "Physical Activity and Depression: Evidence from the Alameda County Study." *Am J Epidemiol* 134(2) (1991):220–231. Paffenbarger, R. S. Jr., I. M. Lee, R. Leung. "Physical Activity and Personal Characteristics Associated with Depression and Suicide in American College Men." *Acta Psychiatr Scand Suppl* 377 (1994):16–22.

58. Blumenthal, J., M. A. Babyak, K. A. Moore, et al. "Effect of Exercise Training on Older Patients with Major Depression." *Arch Intern Med* 159(19) (Oct 25 1999): 2349–2356.

59. Babyak, M., J. Blumenthal, S. Herman, et al. "Exercise Treatment for Major Depression: Maintenance of Therapeutic Benefit at 10 Months." *Psychosom Med* 62(5) (Sep-Oct 2000):633–638.

60. Lawlor, D. A., A. W. Hopker. "The Effectiveness of Exercise as an Intervention in the Management of Depression: Systematic Review and Meta-Regression Analysis of Randomized Controlled Trials." *BMJ* 322(7289) (Mar 31, 2001):763–767. Mead, G. E., W. Morley, P. Campbell, et al. "Exercise for Depression." *Cochrane Database Syst Rev* (Oct 8, 2008) CD004366.

61. Gellner, E. *Plough, Sword and Book: The Structure of Human History.* Chicago: University of Chicago Press, 1988.

62. Cohen, M. N. *Health and the Rise of Civilization.* New Haven: Yale University Press, 1989.

63. Bloom, H. "Instant Evolution. The Influence of the City on Human Genes: A Speculative Case." *New Ideas Psychol* 19(3) (Dec 2001):203–220.

64. Bhugra, D., A. Mastrogianni. "Globalisation and Mental Disorders. Overview with Relation to Depression." *Br J Psychiatry* 184(1) (Jan 2004):10–20.

65. Sundquist, K., G. Frank, J. Sundquist. "Urbanisation and Incidence of Psychosis and Depression: Follow-Up Study of 4.4 Million Women and Men in Sweden." *Br J Psychiatry* 184(4) (Apr 2004):293–298.

66. Kraut, R., M. Patterson, V. Lundmark, et al. "Internet Paradox. A Social Technol-

ogy that Reduces Social Involvement and Psychological Well-Being?" *Am Psychologist* 53(9) (Sep 1998):1017–1031.

67. Castells, M. *The Rise of the Network Society.* 2nd Edition. Oxford: Blackwell Publishers, 2000.

68. Karasek, R., T. Theorell. *Healthy Work: Stress, Productivity, and the Reconstruction of Working Life.* New York: Basic Books, 1990.

69. Dissanayake, E. *What is Art For?* Seattle: University of Washington Press, 1988.

70. Grinde, B. *Darwinian Happiness: Evolution as a Guide for Living and Understanding Human Behavior.* Princeton: Darwin Press, 2002.

71. Botti, S., C. K. Hsee. "Dazed and Confused by Choice: How the Temporal Costs of Choice Freedom Lead to Undesirable Outcomes." *Org Behav Hum Decis Process* 112(2) (July 2010):161–171.

72. Roberts, S., N. J. Temple. "Medical Research: A Bettor's Guide." *Am J Prev Med* 23(3) (Oct 2002):231–232.

73. Jorm, A.F., H. Christensen, K. M. Griffiths, et al. "Effectiveness of Complementary and Self-Help Treatments for Depression." *Med J Aust* 176 Suppl (May 20 2002): S84–96. Manber, R., J. J. B. Allen, M. M. Morris. "Alternative Treatments for Depression: Empirical Support and Relevance to Women." *J Clin Psychiatry* 63(7) (Jul 2002) :628–640.

74. Jorm, A. F., A. E. Korten, P. A. Jacomb, et al. "Helpfulness of Interventions for Mental Disorders: Beliefs of Health Professionals Compared with the General Public." *Br J Psychiatry* 171(3) (Sep 1997):233–237.

75. Sin, N. L., S. Lyubomirsky. "Enhancing Well-Being and Alleviating Depressive Symptoms with Positive Psychology Interventions: A Practice-Friendly Meta-Analysis." *J Clin Psychol* 65(5) (2009):467–487.

76. Wood, A. M., S. Joseph. "The Absence of Positive Psychological (Eudemonic) Well-Being as a Risk Factor for Depression: A Ten Year Cohort Study." *J Affect Dis* 122(3) (May 2010):213–217.

Chapter 3: Conventional Treatment and Traditional Science

1. Frances, A. "Antidepressants Use Skyrockets." *Psychol Today* DSM5 in Distress blog, October 28, 2011. http://www.psychologytoday.com/blog/dsm5-in-distress/201110/antidepressant-use-skyrockets (accessed July 2012).

2. Fava, G. A., E. Offidani. "The Mechanisms of Tolerance in Antidepressant Action." *Prog Neuropsychopharmacol Biol Psychiatry* 35(7) (Aug 15, 2011):1593–1602.

3. Andrews, P. W., S. G. Kornstein, L. J. Halberstadt, et al. "Blue Again: Perturbational Effects of Antidepressants Suggest Monoaminergic Homeostasis in Major Depression." *Front Psychol* 2(159) (2011):1–24.

4. Bolwig, T. G. "How Does Electroconvulsive Therapy Work? Theories on Its Mechanism." *Can J Psychiatry* 56(1) (Jan 2011):13–18.

5. Sackheim, H. A., J. Prudic, R. Fuller, et al. "The Cognitive Effects of Electroconvulsive Therapy in Community Settings." *Neuropsychopharmacology* 32(1) (2007):244–254.

6. Linton, C. R., M. T. P. Reynolds, N. J. Warner. "Using Thiamine to Reduce Post-ECT Confusion." *Int J Geriatr Psychiatry* 17(2) (Feb 2002):189–192.

7. Gould, J. "The Use of Vitamins in Psychiatric Practice." *Proc R Soc Med* 47(3) (Mar 1954):215–220.

8. Gardner, A., R. G. Boles. "Beyond the Serotonin Hypothesis: Mitochondria, Inflammation and Neurodegeneration in Major Depression and Affective Spectrum Disorders." *Prog Neuropsychopharmacol Biol Psychiatry* 35(3) (Apr 29, 2011):730–743.

9. Chalabi, N., D. J. Bernard-Gallon, M. Vasson. "Nutrigenomics and Antioxidants." *Personalized Med* 5(1) (Jan 2008):25–36.

10. Miller, D. W., C. G. Miller. "On Evidence, Medical and Legal." *J Am Phys Surg* 10(3) (2005):70–75.

11. Feinstein, A. R. "Basic Biomedical Science and the Destruction of the Pathophysiologic Bridge from Bench to Bedside." *Am J Med* 107(5) (Nov 1999):461–467.

12. Vincent, J. L. "We Should Abandon Randomized Controlled Trials in the Intensive Care Unit." *Crit Care Med* 38(10 Suppl) (Oct 2010):S534-S538. Salander, P. "It's Futile to Believe that RCT Studies Will Steer Us to Godot." *Psycho-Oncology* 20(3) (Mar 2011):333–334. Kaplan, B., G. Giesbrecht, S. Shannon, et al. "Evaluating Treatments in Health Care: The Instability of a One-Legged Stool." *BMC Med Res Methodol* 11(65) (2011):1–7.

13. Zimmerman, M., J. I. Mattia, M. A. Posternak. "Are Subjects in Pharmacological Treatment Trials of Depression Representative of Patients in Routine Practice?" *Am J Psychiatry* 159(3) (Mar 2002):469–473. Zetin, M., C. Hoepner. "Relevance of Exclusion Criteria in Antidepressant Clinical Trials: A Replication Study." *J Clin Psychopharmacol* 27(3) (Jun 2007):295–301.

14. Patterson, S., K. Kramo, T. Soteriou, et al. "The Great Divide: A Qualitative Investigation of Factors Influencing Researcher Access to Potential Randomized Controlled Trial Participants in Mental Health Settings." *J Ment Health* 19(6) (Dec 2010):532–541.

15. Melander, H., T. Salmonson, E. Abadie, et al. "A Regulatory Apologia–A Review of Placebo-Controlled Studies in Regulatory Submissions of New-Generation Antidepressants." *Eur Neuropsychopharmacol* 18(9) (Sep 2008):623–627.

16. Ioannidis, J. P. "Why Most Published Research Findings Are False." *PLoS Med* 2(8) (2005): e124.

17. Beecher, H. K. "The Powerful Placebo." *JAMA* 159(17) (Dec 24, 1955): 1602–1606.

18. Kienle, G. S., Kiene, H. "The Powerful Placebo Effect: Fact or Fiction?" *J Clin Epidemiol* 50(12) (Dec 1997):1311–1318.

19. Shorter, E. "A Brief History of Placebos and Clinical Trials in Psychiatry." *Can J Psychiatry* 56(4) (Apr 2011):193–197.

20. Golomb, B. A., L. C. Erickson, S. Koperski, et al. "What's in Placebos: Who Knows? Analysis of Randomized, Controlled Trials." *Ann Intern Med* 153(8) (Oct 19, 2010):532–535.

21. Hoffer, A., H. Osmond, M. J. Callbeck, et al. "Treatment of Schizophrenia with Nicotinic acid and Nicotinamide." *J Clin Exp Psychopathol* 18(2) (Aug 15, 1957):131–

158. Hoffer, A. *Adventures in Psychiatry: The Scientific Memoirs of Dr Abram Hoffer.* Caledon, ONT: KOS Publishing, 2005.

22. Hoffer, A. "An Examination of the Double-Blind Method as It Has Been Applied to Megavitamin Therapy." *J Orthomol Psychiatry* 2(3) (1973):107–114.

23. Roberts, L. W., J. Lauriello, C. Geppert, et al. "Placebos and Paradoxes in Psychiatric Research: An Ethics Perspective." *Biol Psychiatry* 49(11) (Jun 1, 2001):887–893.

24. Shapiro, S. "Meta-Analysis/Shmeta-Analysis" *Am J Epidemiol* 140(9) (Nov 1, 1994):771–778. Moayyedi, P. "Meta-Analysis: Can We Mix Apples and Oranges?" *Am J Gastroenterol* 99(12) (Dec 2004):2297–2301. Ioannidis, J. P., T. A. Trikalinos. "The Appropriateness of Asymmetry Tests for Publication Bias in Meta-Analyses: A Large Survey." *Can Med Assoc J* 176(8) (Apr 10, 2007):1091–1096.

25. Miller, E. R. 3rd, R. Pastor-Barriuso, D. Dalal, et al. "Meta-Analysis: High-Dosage Vitamin E Supplementation May Increase All-Cause Mortality." *Ann Intern Med* 142(1) (Jan 4, 2005):37–46. Bjelakovic, G., D. Nikolova, L. L. Gluud, et al. "Mortality in Randomized Trials of Antioxidant Supplements for Primary and Secondary Prevention: Systematic Review and Meta-Analysis." *JAMA* 297(8) (Feb 28, 2007):842–857.

26. Hickey, S., L. Noriegai, H. Roberts. "Poor Methodology in Meta-Analysis of Vitamins." *J Orthomol Med* 22(1) (2007):8–10.

27. Biesalski, H. K., T. Grune, J. Tinz, et al. "Reexaminatioon of a Meta-Analysis of the Effect of Antioxidant Supplementation on Mortality and Health in Randomized Trials." *Nutrients* 2(9) (2010):929–949.

28. Melander, H., J. Ahlqvist-Rastad, G. Meijer, et al. "Evidence B(i)ased Medicine— Selective Reporting from Studies Sponsored by Pharmaceutical Industry: Review of Studies in New Drug Applications." *BMJ* 326(7400) (May 29, 2003):1171–1173. Turner, E. H., A. M. Matthews, E. Linardatos, et al. "Selective Publication of Antidepressant Trials and Its Influence on Apparent Efficacy." *New Engl J Med* 358(3) (Jan 17, 2008):252–260.

29. Horrobin, D. F. "The Philosophical Basis of Peer Review and the Suppression of Innovation." *JAMA* 263(10) (Mar 9, 1990):1438–1441. Rothwell, P. M., C. N. Martyn. "Reproducibility of Peer Review in Clinical Neuroscience. Is Agreement between Reviewers Any Greater than Would Be Expected by Chance Alone?" *Brain* 123(9) (2000):1964–1969. Horrobin, D. F. "Something Rotten at the Core of Science?" *Trends Pharmacol Sci* 22(2) (Feb 2001):51–52. Smith, R. "Peer Review: A Flawed Process at the Heart of Science and Journals." *J R Soc Med* 99(4) (Apr 2006)178–182. Smith, R. "Classical Peer Review: An Empty Gun." *Breast Cancer Res* 12(Suppl 4) (2010):S13.

30. Fanelli, D. "How Many Scientists Fabricate and Falsify Research? A Systematic Review and Meta-Analysis of Survey Data." *PLoS One* 4(5) (May 29, 2009):e5738. Michalek, A. M., A. D. Hutson, C. P. Wicher, et al. "The Costs and Underappreciated Consequences of Research Misconduct: A Case Study." *PLoS Med* 7(8) (Aug 17, 2010):e1000318.

31. Gotzsche, P. C., A. Hróbjartsson, H. K. Johansen, et al. "Ghost Authorship in Industry-Initiated Randomised Trials." *PLoS Med* 4(1) (Jan 2007):e19. Sismondo, S. "Ghost Management: How Much of the Medical Literature Is Shaped Behind the Scenes by the Pharmaceutical Industry?" *PLoS Med* 4(9) (Sep 2007):e286. Barbour,

V. "How Ghost-Writing Threatens the Credibility of Medical Knowledge and Medical Journals." *Haematologica* 95(1) (Jan 2010):1–2.

32. Lacasse, J. R., J. Leo. "Ghostwriting at Elite Academic Medical Centers in the United States." *PLoS Med* 7(2) (Feb 2, 2010):e1000230.

33. Wislar, J. S., A. Flanagin, P. B. Fontanarosa, et al. "Honorary and Ghost Authorship in High Impact Biomedical Journals: A Cross Sectional Survey." *BMJ* 343 (Oct 25, 2011):d6128.

34. Resnik, D. B. *The Price of Truth: How Money Affects the Norms of Science.* New York: Oxford University Press, 2007.

35. Platt, J. R. "Diversity." *Science* 154(3753) (Dec 2, 1966):1132–1139.

36. Krimsky, S., L. S. Rothenberg. "Financial Interest and Its Discosure in Scientific Publications." *JAMA* 280(3) (Jul 15, 1998):225–226. Angell, M. *The Truth About the Drug Companies: How They Deceive Us and What to Do About It.* New York: Random House, 2004. Smith, R. "Medical Journals Are an Extension of the Marketing Arm of Pharmaceutical Companies." *PLoS Med* 2(5) (May 2005):e138. Smith, R. *The Trouble with Medical Journals.* London: Royal Society Medicine Press, 2006.

37. Sismondo, S. "How Pharmaceutical Industry Funding Affects Trial Outcomes: Causal Structures and Responses." *Soc Sci Med* 66(9) (May 2008):1909–1914.

38. Lesser, L. I., C. B. Ebbeling, M. Goozner, et al. "Relationship between Funding Source and Conclusion among Nutrition-Related Scientific Articles." *PLoS Med* 4(1) (Jan 2007): e5.

39. Starcevic, V. "Opportunistic 'Rediscovery' of Mental Disorders by the Pharmaceutical Industry." *Psychother Psychosom* 71(6) (Nov-Dec 2002):305–310.

40. Lane, C. *Shyness: How Normal Behavior Became a Sickness.* New Haven: Yale University Press, 2007.

41. Horwitz, A. V., J. C. Wakefield. *The Loss of Sadness: How Psychiatry Transformed Normal Sorrow into Depressive Disorder.* New York: Oxford University Press, 2007.

42. Cosgrove, L., S. Krimsky, M. Vijayaraghavan, et al. "Financial Ties between DSM-IV Panel Members and the Pharmaceutical Industry." *Psychother Psychosom* 75(3) (2006):154–160. Cosgrove, L., H. J. Bursztajn, S. Krimsky, et al. "Conflicts of Interest and Disclosure in the American Psychiatric Association's Clinical Practice Guidelines." *Psychother Psychosom* 78(4) (2009):228–232.

43. Horrobin, D. F. *Science Is God.* Aylesbury (Bucks): Medical and Technical Publishing, 1969.

44. Clerc, O. *Modern Medicine: The New World Religion—How Beliefs Secretly Influence Medical Dogmas and Practices.* Fawnskin, CA: Personhood Press, 2004.

45. Riordan, H.D. "Book Reviews [Review of the book *Ascorbate: The Science of Vitamin C*]." *J Orthomol Med* 20(2nd Quarter) (2005):123.

46. Evidence-Based Medicine Working Group. "Evidence-Based Medicine. A New Approach to Teaching the Practice of Medicine." *JAMA* 268(17) (Nov 4, 1992):2420–2425.

47. Straus, S. E., P. Glasziou, W. S. Richardson, et al. *Evidence-Based Medicine: How to Practice and Teach It.* 4th edition. London: Churchill Livingstone, 2011.

48. Stahl, S. M. "Antipsychotic Polypharmacy: Evidence Based or Eminence Based? *Acta Psychiatr Scand* 106(5) (Nov 2002):321–322. Rosner, A. L. "Evidence-Based Medicine: Revisiting the Pyramid of Priorities." *J Bodyw Mov Ther* 16(1) (Jan 2012):42–49.

Chapter 4: Evidence-Based Medicine: Neither Good Evidence nor Good Medicine

1. Hickey, S., H. Roberts. *Tarnished Gold: The Sickness of Evidence-Based Medicine.* CreateSpace, 2011.

2. Vandenbroucke, J. P. "Observational Research, Randomised Trials, and Two Views of Medical Science." *PLoS Med* 5(3) (Mar 11, 2008):e67.

Chapter 5: Orthomolecular Medicine and Biochemical Individuality

1. Pauling, L. "Orthomolecular Psychiatry." *Molecular Medicine* (1967):1–6.

2. Pauling, L. "Orthomolecular Psychiatry: Varying the Concentrations of Substances Normally Present in the Human Body May Control Mental Disease." *Science* 160(3825) (Apr 19, 1968):265–271.

3. Blumberg, J., R. P. Heaney, M. Huncharek, et al. "Evidence-Based Criteria in the Nutritional Context." *Nutr Rev* 68(8) (Aug 2010):478–484. Shao, A., Mackay, D. "A Commentary on the Nutrient-Chronic Disease Relationship and the New Paradigm of Evidence-Based Nutrition." *Natural Med J* 2(12) (Dec 1, 2010):10–18.

4. Bruder, C. E., A. Piotrowski, A. A. Gijsbers, et al. "Phenotypically Concordant and Discordant Monozygotic Twins Display Different DNA Copy-Number-Variation Profiles." *Am J Hum Genet* 82(3) (Mar 2008):763–771.

5. Bearn, A. G. *Archibald Garrod and the Individuality of Man.* Oxford: Clarendon Press, 1993.

6. Garrod, A. E. "The Incidence of Alkaptonuria: A Study in Chemical Individuality." *Lancet* 160(4137) (1902):1616–1620.

7. Williams, R. J. *Biochemical Individuality.* New Canaan, CT: Keats, 1998.

8. Zhao, J. "Genomic Individuality and Its Biological Implications." *Med Hypothes* 46(6) (Jun 1996):499–502.

9. Widdowson, E. M. "Nutritional individuality." *Proc Nutr Soc* 21(2) (1962):121–128. Eckhardt, R. B. "Genetic Research and Nutritional Individuality." *J Nutr* 131(2) (Feb 2001):336S–339S.

Chapter 6: An Evolution-Based Health Program

1. Hedaya, R. J. *The Antidepressant Survival Guide.* New York: Three Rivers Press, 2000.

2. Servan-Schreiber, D. *Healing Without Freud or Prozac: Natural Approaches to Curing Stress, Anxiety and Depression,* Revised ed. London: Rodale, 2005.

3. Ilardi, S. S. *The Depression Cure: The 6-Step Program to Beat Depression without Drugs.* Cambridge, MA: Da Capo Press, 2009.

4. Barsky, A. J., E. C. Deans. *Feeling Better: A 6-Week Mind-Body Program to Ease Your Chronic Symptoms.* New York: Collins, 2007.

5. Whalen, R. "Caffeine Allergy: Past Disorder or Present Epidemic?" DoctorYourself .com, (2001). http://www.doctoryourself.com/caffeine_allergy.html (accessed July 2012). Whalen, R. *Welcome to the Dance: Caffeine Allergy—A Masked Cerebral Allergy and Progressive Toxic Dementia.* Victoria, BC: Trafford Publishing, 2006.

Chapter 7: Food Really Does Matter

1. Wahlqvist, M. L. "'Malnutrition' in the Aged: The Dietary Assessment." *Public Health Nutrition* 5(6A) (Dec 2002):911–913. Delisle, H. F. "Poverty: The Double Burden of Malnutrition in Mothers and the Intergenerational Impact." *Ann N Y Acad Sci* 1136 (2008):172–184.

2. Sonestedt, E., C. Roos, B. Gullberg, et al. "Fat and Carbohydrate Intake Modify the Association between Genetic Variation in the *FTO* Genotype and Obesity." *Am J Clin Nutr* 90(5) (Sep 2, 2009):1418–1425.

3. Cornier, M. A., W. T. Donahoo, R. Pereira, et al. "Insulin Sensitivity Determines the Effectivemness of Dietary Macronutrient Composition on Weight Loss in Obese Women." *Obes Res* 13(4) (Apr 2005):703–709.

4. Westover, A. N., L. B. Marangell. "A Cross-National Relationship between Sugar Consumption and Major Depression?" *Depress Anxiety* 16(3) (2002):118–120. Peet, M. "International Variations in the Outcome of Schizophrenia and the Prevalence of Depression in Relation to National Dietary Practices: An Ecological Analysis." *Br J Psychiatry* 184(5) (May 2004):404–408.

5. Lien, L., N. Lien, S. Heyerdahl, et al. "Consumption of Soft Drinks and Hyperactivity, Mental Distress, and Conduct Problems among Adolescents in Oslo, Norway." *Am J Publ Health* 96(10) (Oct 2006):1815–1820.

6. Golomb, B. A., L. Tenkanen, T. Alikoski, et al. "Insulin Sensitivity Markers: Predictors of Accidents and Suicides in Helsinki Heart Study Screenees." *J Clin Epidem* 55(8) (Aug 2002):767–773.

7. Lawlor, D. A., G. D. Smith, S. Ebrahim. "Association of Insulin Resistance with Depression: Cross Sectional Findings from the British Women's Heart and Health Study." *BMJ* 327(7428) (Dec 13, 2003):1383–1384.

8. Sánchez-Villegas, A., M. Delgado-Rodríguez, A. Alonso, et al. "Association of the Mediterranean Dietary Pattern with the Incidence of Depression: the Seguimiento Universidad de Navarra/University of Navarra Follow-Up (SUN) Cohort." *Arch Gen Psychiatry* 66(10) (Oct 2009):1090–1098.

9. Akbaraly, T. N., E. J. Brunner, J. E. Ferrie, et al. "Dietary Pattern and Depressive Symptoms in Middle Age." *Br J Psychiatry* 195(5) (Nov 2009):408–413.

10. Jacka, F. N., J. A. Pasco, A. Mykletun, et al. "Association of Western and Traditional Diets with Depression and Anxiety in Women." *Am J Psychiatry* 167(3) (Mar 2010):305–311.

11. Jacka, F. N., P. J. Kremer, M. Berk, et al. "A Prospective Study of Diet Quality and Mental Health in Adolescents." *PLoS One* 6(9) (Sep 21, 2011): e24805.

12. Gelenberg, A. J., J. D. Wojcik, J. H. Growdon, et al. "Tyrosine for the Treatment of Depression," *American Journal of Psychiatry*, 1347(5):622, (May, 1980) 622–623.

13. "Lecithin and Memory." *Lancet* 1(8163) (Feb 9, 1980):293.

14. "Choline and Lecithin for a Better Memory." *Today's Living* (February 1982).

Chapter 8: Orthomolecular Treatment

1. Machlin, L. J. "Introduction." *Ann N Y Acad Sci* 669 (Dec 17, 1992):1–6.

2. Altschul, R., A. Hoffer, J. D. Stephen. "Influence of Nicotinic Acid on Serum Cholesterol in Man." *Arch Biochem Biophys* 54(2) (Feb 1955):558–559.

3. Leape, L. L. "Error in Medicine." *JAMA.* 272(23) (Dec 21, 1994):1851–1857. Leape, L. L. "Institute of Medicine Medical Error Figures Are Not Exaggerated." *JAMA* 284(1) (Jul 5, 2000):95–7.

4. Dean, C., M. Feldman, D. Rasio, et al. "Death by Medicine." DoctorYourself.com, (December 2003). http://www.doctoryourself.com/deathmed.html (accessed July 2012).

5. Klein, E. A., I. M. Thompson, C. M. Tangen, et al. "Vitamin E and the Risk of Prostate Cancer: The Selenium and Vitamin E Cancer Prevention Trial (SELECT)." *JAMA.* 306(14) (Oct 12, 2011):1549–1556. http://jama.ama-assn.org/content/306/ 14/1549 (accessed July 2012).

6. Orthomolecular.org. "Rigged Trials: Drug Studies Favor the Manufacturer." Orthomolecular Medicine News Service. November 5, 2008. http://orthomolecular.org/ resources/omns/v04n20.shtml (accessed July 2012).

7. Orthomolecular.org. "Pharmaceutical Advertising Biases Journals Against Vitamin Supplements." Orthomolecular Medicine News Service. February 5, 2009. http://ortho-molecular.org/resources/omns/v05n02.shtml (accessed July 2012).

8. Orthomolecular.org. "NLM Censors Nutritional Research." Orthomolecular Medicine News Service. January 15, 2010. http://orthomolecular.org/resources/omns/v06n03. shtml (accessed July 2012). Orthomolecular.org. "How to Fool All of the People All of the Time." Orthomolecular Medicine News Service. January 21, 2010. http://orthomolecular. org/ resources/omns/v06n05.shtml (accessed July 2012).

9. Fawzi, W. W., G. I. Msamanga, D. Spiegelman, et al. "A Randomized Trial of Multivitamin Supplements and HIV Disease Progression and Mortality. *N Engl J Med* 351(1) (Jul 1, 2004):23–32.

10. Orthomolecular.org. "No Deaths from Vitamins: America's Largest Database Confirms Supplement Safety." Orthomolecular Medicine News Service, December 28, 2011 http://orthomolecular.org/resources/omns/v07n16.shtml (accessed Aug 2012).

11. Associated Press. "Bad Drug Reactions Send 700,000 to ER Yearly." msnbc.com Health Care. Oct 17, 2006. http://www.msnbc.msn.com/id/15305033/ (accessed July 2012).

12. Null, G., C. Dean, M. Feldman, et al. "Death by Medicine." *J Orthomolecular Med.* 20(1) (2005):21–34. Available online at: http://orthomolecular.org/library/jom/ 2005/pdf/2005-v20n01-p021.pdf or http://www.doctoryourself.com/deathmed.html. Further discussion in: Dean, C., T. Tuck. *Death by Modern Medicine.* Belleville, ON: Matrix Verite, 2005.

13. Associated Press. "Drug Errors Injure More than 1.5 Million a Year." msnbc.com

Health Care. July 20, 2006. http://www.msnbc.msn.com/id/13954142 (accessed July 2012).

14. Leape, L. L. "Institute of Medicine Medical Error Figures Are Not Exaggerated." *JAMA* 284(1) (Jul 5, 2000):95–7. Leape, L. L. "Error in Medicine." *JAMA* 272(23) (Dec 21, 1994):1851–7. Lazarou, J., B. H. Pomeranz, P. N. Corey. "Incidence of Adverse Drug Reactions in Hospitalized Patients: A Meta-Analysis of Prospective Studies." *JAMA* 279(15) (Apr 15, 1998):1200–5.

15. Bayer Healthcare. "Expect Wonders." http://www.wonderdrug.com/ (formerly http://www.bayeraspirin.com/news/heart_attack.htm) (accessed July 2012).

16. Reuters. "Daily Aspirin Use Linked with Pancreatic Cancer." CNN.com/Health. (Oct 27, 2003) http://www.cnn.com/2003/HEALTH/10/27/cancer.aspirin.reut/index .html (accessed July 2012).

17. Brozek, J. "Psychologic Effects of Thiamine Restriction and Deprivation in Normal Young Men." *Am J Clin Nutr* 5(2) (1957):109–120.

18. Smidt, L. J., F. M. Cremin, L. E. Grivetti, et al. "Influence of Thiamin Supplementation on the Health and General Well-Being of an Elderly Irish Population with Marginal Thiamin Deficiency." *J Gerontol* 46(1) (Jan 1991):M16–M22.

19. Benton, D., J. Haller, J. Fordy. "Vitamin Supplementation for 1 Year Improves Mood." *Neuropsychobiology* 32(2) (1995):98–105.

20. Benton, D., R. Griffiths, J. Haller. "Thiamine Supplementation, Mood and Cognitive Functioning." *Psychopharmacology (Berl)* 129(1) (Jan 1997):66–71.

21. Sterner, R. T., W. R. Price. "Restricted Riboflavin: Within-Subject Behavioral Effects in Humans." *Am J Clin Nutr* 26(2) (Feb 1973):150–160.

22. Carney, M. W. P., A. Ravindran, M. G. Rinsler, et al. "Thiamine, Riboflavin and Pyridoxine Deficiency in Psychiatric In-Patients." *Br J Psychiat* 141 (Sep 1982): 271–272.

23. Benton, D., J. Haller, J. Fordy. "Vitamin Supplementation for 1 Year Improves Mood." *Neuropsychobiology* 32(2) (1995):98–105.

24. Berger, F., M. H. Ramírez-Hernández, M. Ziegler. "The New Life of a Centenarian: Signalling Functions of NAD(P)." *Trends Biochem Sci* 29(3) (Mar 2004):111–118. Billington, R. A., S. Bruzzone, A. De Flora, et al. "Emerging Functions of Extracellular Pyridine Nucleotides." *Mol Med* 12(11–12) (Nov-Dec 2006):324–327. Koch-Nolte, F., F. Haag, A. H Guse, et al. "Emerging Roles of NAD+ and Its Metabolites in Cell Signaling." *Sci Signal* 2(57) (Feb 10, 2009):mr1.

25. Imai, S. "'Clocks' in the NAD World: NAD as a Metabolic Oscillator for the Regulation of Metabolism and Aging." *Biochim Biophys Acta* 1804(8) (Aug 2010): 1584–1590.

26. Li, F., Z. Z. Chong, K. Maiese. "Navigating Novel Mechanisms of Cellular Plasticity with the NAD+ Precursor and Nutrient Nicotinamide." *Front Biosci* 9 (Sep 1, 2004):2500–2520.

27. Hoffer, A., H. D. Foster. *Feel Better, Live Longer with Vitamin B₃: Nutrient Deficiency and Dependency.* Toronto: CCNM Press, 2007. Bogan, K. L., C. Brenner. "Nic-

otinic Acid, Nicotinamide, and Nicotinamide Riboside: A Molecular Evaluation of NAD+ Precursor Vitamins in Human Nutrition." *Annu Rev Nutr* 28 (2008):115–130.

28. Hawkins, D., L. Pauling. *Orthomolecular Psychiatry: Treatment of Schizophrenia.* San Francisco: W. H. Freeman, 1973.

29. Hoffer, A., A. W. Saul, H. D. Foster. *Niacin: The Real Story.* Laguna Beach, CA: Basic Health Publications, 2011.

30. Altschul, R., A. Hoffer, J. D. Stephen. "Influence of Nicotinic Acid on Serum Cholesterol in Man." *Arch Biochem Biophys* 54(2) (Feb 1955):558–559.

31. Ungerstedt, J. S., M. Blömback, T. Söderström. "Nicotinamide Is a Potent Inhibitor of Proinflammatory Cytokines." *Clin Expo Immunol* 131(1) (Jan 2003):48–52.

32. Kaufman, W. *The Common Form of Joint Dysfunction: Its Incidence and Treatment.* Brattleboro, VT: Hildreth & Co, 1949.

33. Jonas, W. B., C. P. Rapoza, W. F. Blair. "The Effect of Niacinamide on Osteoarthritis: A Pilot Study." *Inflamm Res* 45(7) (Jul 1996):330–334.

34. Hoffer, A., H. Osmond, M. J. Callbeck, et al. "Treatment of Schizophrenia with Nicotinic Acid and Nicotinamide." *J Clin Exp Psychopathol* 18(2) (Apr-Jun 1957):131–158. Osmond, H., A. Hoffer. "Massive Niacin Treatment in Schizophrenia. Review of a Nine-Year Study." *Lancet* 7224 (1962): 316–320.

35. Miller, C. L., J. R. Dulay. "The High-Affinity Receptor HM74A Is Decreased in the Anterior Cingulated Cortex of Individuals with Schizophrenia." *Brain Res Bull* 77(1) (Sep 5, 2008):33–41.

36. Möhler, H., P. Polc, R. Cumin, et al. "Nicotinamide Is a Brain Constituent with Benzodiazepine-Like Actions." *Nature* 278(5704) (Apr 5, 1979):563–565. Tallman, J. F., S. M. Paul, P. Skolnick, et al. "Receptors for the Age of Anxiety: Pharmacology of the Benzodiazepines." *Science* 207(4428) (Jan 18, 1980):274–281.

37. Vescovi, P. P., G. Gerra, L. Ippolito, et al. "Nicotinic Acid Effectiveness in the Treatment of Benzodiazepine Withdrawal." *Curr Ther Res* 41(6) (1987):1017–1021.

38. Babcock, J. W. "The Prevalence and Psychology of Pellagra." *Am J Insanity* 67(3) (1911):517–540. Spies, T. G., C. D. Aring, J. Gelperin, et al. "The Mental Symptoms of Pellagra: Their Relief with Nicotinic Acid." *Am J Med Sci* 196(4) (Oct 1938):461–475. Aring, C. D., T. D. Spies. "A Critical Review: Vitamin B Deficiency and Nervous Disease." *J Neurol Psychiatry* 2(4) (Oct 1939):335–360.

39. Washburne, A. C. "Nicotinic Acid in the Treatment of Certain Depressed States: A Preliminary Report." *Ann Intern Med* 32(2) (Feb 1950):261–269.

40. Tonge, W. L. "Nicotinic Acid in the Treatment of Depression." *Ann Intern Med* 38(3) (Mar 1, 1953) 551–553.

41. Malcolm, R. "Nicotinic Acid and Depression: Depression Following Cessation of Nicotinic Acid Use." *Psychosomatics* 16(2) (Apr 1975):68–69.

42. Chouinard, G., S. N. Young, L. Annable, et al. "Tryptophan-Nicotinamide, Imipramine and Their Combination in Depression. A Controlled Study." *Acta Psychiatr Scand* 59(4) (Apr 1979):395–414.

43. Prousky, J. E. "Vitamin B_3 for Depression: Case Report and Review of the Literature." *J Orthomol Med* 25(3) (2010):137–147.

44. Birkmayer, G. D. *NADH: The Biological Hydrogen: The Secret of Our Life Energy.* Laguna Beach, CA: Basic Health Publications, 2009.

45. Birkmayer, J. G. D., W. Birkmayer. "The Coenzyme Nicotinamide Adenine Dinucleotide (NADH) as Biological Antidepressive Agent: Experience with 205 Patients." *New Trends Clin Neuropharmacol* 5(314) (1991):75–86.

46. Ebadi, M. "Regulation and Function of Pyridoxal Phosphate in CNS." *Neurochem Int* 3(3–4) (1981):181–205.

47. Clayton, P. T. "B_6-Responsive Disorders: A Model of Vitamin Dependency." *J Inherit Metab Dis* 29(2–3) (Apr–Jun 2006):317–326.

48. Dalton, K., M. J. Dalton. "Characteristics of Pyridoxine Overdose Neuropathy Syndrome." *Acta Neurol Scand* 76(1) (Jul 1987):8–11.

49. Holford, P., S. Heaton. "Vitamin B_6: Extract of Submission to the UK's Food Standards Agency." *J Orthomol Med* 18(3–4) (2003):161–165.

50. Bender, D. A. "Non-Nutritional Uses of Vitamin B_6." *Br J Nutr* 81(1) (Jan 1999):7–20.

51. Murakami, K., Y. Miyake, S. Sasaki, "Dietary Folate, Riboflavin, Vitamin B_6, and Vitamin B_{12} and Depressive Symptoms in Early Adolescence: The Ryukyus Child Health Study." *Psychosom Med* 72(8) (Oct 2010):763–768.

52. Williams, A. L., A. Cotter, A. Sabina, et al. "The Role for Vitamin B_6 as Treatment for Depression: A Systematic Review." *Fam Pract* 22(5) (Oct 2005):532–537.

53. Coppen, A., J. Bailey. "Enhancement of the Antidepressant Action of Fluoxetine by Folic Acid: A Randomized, Placebo Controlled Trial." *J Affect Disord* 60(2) (Nov 2000):121–130.

54. Coppen, A., G. Bolander-Gouaille. "Treatment of Depression: Time to Consider Folic Acid and Vitamin B_{12}." *J Psychopharmacol* 19(1) (Jan 2005):59–65.

55. Abou-Saleh, M. T., A. Coppen. "Folic Acid and the Treatment of Depression." *J Psychosom Res* 61(3) (Sep 2006):285–287.

56. Stahl, S. M. "L-Methylfolate: A Vitamin for Your Monoamines." *J Clin Psychiatry* 69(9) (Sep 2008):1352–1353.

57. Hodgkin, D. C., J. Kamper, M. MacKay, et al. "Structure of Vitamin B_{12}." *Nature* 178(4524) (Jul 14, 1956):64–66.

58. Bottiglieri, T. "Folate, Vitamin B_{12}, and Neuropsychiatric Disorders." *Nutr Rev* 54(12) (Dec 1996):382–390.

59. Birch, C. S., N. E. Brasch, A. McCaddon, et al. "A Novel Role for Vitamin B_{12}: Cobalamins Are Intracellular Antioxidants In Vitro." *Free Radic Biol Med* 47(2) (Jul 15, 2009):184–188.

60. Lindenbaum, J., E. B. Healton, D. G. Savage, et al. "Neuropsychiatric Disorders Caused by Cobalamin Deficiency in the Absence of Anemia or Macrocytosis." *New Engl J Med* 318(26) (Jun 30, 1988):1720–1728.

61. Goebels, N., M. Soyka. "Dementia Associated with Vitamin B_{12} Deficiency: Presen-

tation of Two Cases and Review of the Literature." *J Neuropsychiatry Clin Neurosci* 12(3) (Summer 2000):389–394.

62. Bar-Shai, M., D. Gott, S. Marmor. "Acute Psychotic Depression as a Sole Manifestation of Vitamin B$_{12}$ Deficiency." *Psychosomatics* 52(4) (Jul-Aug 2011): 384–386.

63. Pacholok, S. M., J. J. Stuart. *Could It Be B$_{12}$? An Epidemic of Misdiagnosis.* Sanger, CA: Quill Driver Books, 2005.

64. van Tiggelen, C. J., J. P. Peperkamp, J. F. Tertoolen. "Vitamin B$_{12}$ Levels of Cerebrospinal Fluid in Patients with Organic Mental Disorder." *J Orthomol Psychiatry* 12(4) (1983):305–311. van Tiggelen, C. J., J. P. Peperkamp, H. J. Tertoolen. "Assessment of Vitamin B$_{12}$ Status in CSF." *Am J Psychiatry* 141(1) (Jan 1984):136–137.

65. Stanger, O., B. Fowler, K. Pietrzik, et al. "Homocysteine, Folate and Vitamin B$_{12}$ in Neuropsychiatric Diseases: Review and Treatment Recommendations." *Expert Rev Neurother* 9(9) (Sep 2009):1393–1412.

66. Froese, D. S., R. A. Gravel. "Genetic Disorders of Vitamin B$_{12}$ Metabolism: Eight Complementation Groups—Eight Genes." *Expert Rev Mol Med* 12 (Nov 2010):e37.

67. Hintikka, J., T. Tolmunen, A. Tanskanen, et al. "High Vitamin B$_{12}$ Level and Good Treatment Outcome May Be Associated in Major Depressive Disorder." *BMC Psychiatry* 3 (2003):17.

68. Fain, O., J. Pariés, B. Jacquart, et al. "Hypovitaminosis in Hospitalized Patients." *Eur J Intern Med* 14(7) (Nov 2003):419–425. Olmedo, J. M., J. A. Yiannias, E. B. Windgassen, et al. "Scurvy: A Disease Almost Forgotten." *Int J Dermatol* 45(8) (Aug 2006):909–913. Gan, R., S. Eintracht, L. J. Hoffer. "Vitamin C Deficiency in a University Teaching Hospital." *J Am Coll Nutr* 27(3) (Jun 2008):428–433. Velandia, B., R. M. Centor, V. McConnell. "Scurvy Is Still Present in Developed Countries." 23(8) (Aug 2008):1281–1284. Léger, D. "Scurvy. Remergence of Nutritional Deficiencies." *Can Fam Physician* 54(10) (Oct 2008):1403–1406. R. L. Schleicher, M. D. Carroll, E. C. Ford. "Serum Vitamin C and the Prevalence of Vitamin C Deficiency in the United States: 2003–2004 National Health and Nutrition Examination Survey (NHANES)." *Am J Clin Nutr* 90(5) (Nov 2009):1252–1263. Algahtani, H. L., A. P. Abdu, I. M. Khojah, et al. "Inability to Walk Due to Scurvy: A Forgotten Disease." *Ann Saudi Med* 30(4) (Jul–Aug 2010):325–328.

69. Harrison, F. E., J. M. May. "Vitamin C Function in the Brain: Vital Role of the Ascorbate Transporter SVCT2." *Free Radic Bio Med* 46(6) (Mar 15, 2009):719–730.

70. Calero, C. I., E. Vickers, G. M. Cid, et al. "Allosteric Modulation of Retinal GABA Receptors by Ascorbic acid." *J Neurosci* 31(26) (Jun 29, 2011):9672–9682.

71. Mandl, J., A. Szarka, G. Bánhegyi. "Vitamin C: Update on Physiology and Pharmacology." *Br J Pharmacol* 157(7) (Aug 2009):1097–1110.

72. Belin, S., F. Kaya, S. Burtey, et al. "Ascorbic Acid and Gene Expression: Another Example of Regulation of Gene Expression by Small Molecules?" *Curr Genomics* 11(1) (Mar 2010):52–57.

73. Delanghe, J. R., M. R. Langlois, M. L. de Buyzere, et al. "Vitamin C Deficiency: More than Just a Nutritional Disorder." *Genes Nutr* 6(4) (Nov 2011):341–346.

74. Block, G., N. Shaikh, C. D. Jensen, et al. "Serum Vitamin C and Other Biomarkers Differ by Genotype of Phase 2 Enzyme Genes GSTM1 and GSTT1." *Am J Clin Nutr* 94(3) (Sep 2011):929–937.

75. Rivas, C. I., F. A. Zúñiga, A. Salas-Burgos, et al. "Vitamin C Transporters." *J Physiol Biochem* 64(4) (Dec 2008):357–376.

76. Price, K. D., C. S. Price, R. D. Reynolds. "Hyperglycemia-Induced Ascorbic Acid Deficiency Promotes Endothelial Dysfunction and the Development of Atherosclerosis." *Atherosclerosis* 158(1) (Sep 2001):1–12.

77. Brody, S. "High-Dose Ascorbic Acid Increases Intercourse Frequency and Improves Mood: A Randomized Controlled Trial." *Biol Psychiatry* 52(4) (Aug 15, 2002):371–374.

78. Kinsman, R. A., J. Hood. "Some Behavioral Effects of Ascorbic Acid Deficiency." *Am J Clin Nutr* 24(4) (Apr 1971):455–464.

79. Milner, G. "Ascorbic Acid in Chronic Psychiatric Patients—A Controlled Trial." *Br J Psychiatry* 109 (1963):294–299.

80. Zhang, M., L. Robitaille, S. Eintracht, et al. "Vitamin C Provision Improves Mood in Acutely Hospitalized Patients." *Nutrition* 27(5) (May 2011):530–533.

81. Downing, D. *Daylight Robbery: Sunlight—the Ultimate Detoxifier?* London: Arrow Books, 1988. Sorenson, M. *Vitamin D3 and Solar Power.* Volume 2 of *Solar Power for Optimal Health.* 2nd edition. St. George, UT: Dimension Design & Print, 2008. Holick, M. F. *The Vitamin D Solution: A 3-Step Strategy to Cure Our Most Common Health Problem.* London: Hudson Street Press, 2010.

82. McCann, J. C., B. N. Ames. "Is There Convincing Biological or Behavioral Evidence Linking Vitamin D Deficiency to Brain Dysfunction?" *FASEB J* 22(4) (Apr 2008):982–1001.

83. Ubbenhorst, A., S. Striebich, F. Lang, et al. "Exploring the Relationship between Vitamin D and Basic Personality Traits." *Psychopharmacology* 215(4) (Jun 2011): 733–737.

84. Lansdowne, A. T. G., S. C. Provost. "Vitamin D3 Enhances Mood in Healthy Subjects in Winter." *Psychopharmacology (Berl)* 135(4) (Feb 1998):319–323.

85. Gloth, F. M. 3rd, W. Alam, B. Hollis. "Vitamin D vs Broad Spectrum Phototherapy in the Treatment of Seasonal Affective Disorder." *J Nutr Health Aging* 3(1) (1999):5–7.

86. Parker, G., H. Brotchie. "'D' for Depression: Any Role for Vitamin D? 'Food for Thought' II." *Acta Psychiatr Scand* 124(4) (Oct 2011):243–249.

87. Khamba, B. K., M. Aucoin, D. Tsirgielis, et al. "Effectiveness of Vitamin D in the Treatment of Mood Disorders: A Literature Review." *J Orthomol Med* 26(3) (2011):127–135.

88. Wester, P. O. "Magnesium." *Am J Clin Nutr* 45(5 Suppl) (May 1987):1305–1312. Saris, N. E., E. Mervaala, H. Karppanen, et al. "Magnesium. An Update on Physiological, Clinical and Analytical Aspects." *Clin Chim Acta* 294(1–2) (Apr 2000):1–26. Seelig, M., A. Rosanoff. *The Magnesium Factor.* New York: Avery, 2003. Dean, C. *The Magnesium Miracle.* New York: Ballantine Books, 2007. Sircus, M., A. E. Abraham. *Transdermal Magnesium Therapy.* Chandler, AZ: Phaelos Books & Mediawerks,

2007. Torshin, I. Y., O. Gromova. *Magnesium and Pyridoxine: Fundamental Studies and Clinical Practice.* New York: Nova Science Publishers, 2009.

89. Iseri, L. T., J. H. French. "Magnesium: Nature's Physiologic Calcium Blocker." *Am Heart J* 108(1) (Jul 1984):188–193.

90. Zahradnik, I., I. Minarovic, A. Zahradniková. "Inhibition of the Cardiac L-Type Calcium Channel Current by Antidepressant Drugs." *J Pharmacol Exp Ther* 324(3) (Mar 2008):977–984.

91. Lindberg, G., K. Bingefors, J. Ranstam, et al. "Use of Calcium Channel Blockers and Risk of Suicide: Ecological Findings Confirmed in Population Based Cohort Study." *BMJ* 316(7133) (1998):741–745.

92. Banki, C. M., M. Vojnik, Z. Papp, et al. "Cerebrospinal Magnesium and Calcium Related to Amine Metabolites, Diagnosis, and Suicide Attempts." *Biol Psychiatry* 20(2) (Feb 1985):163–171.

93. Levine, J., D. Stein, R. Rapoport, et al. "High Serum and Cerebrospinal Fluid Ca/Mg Ratio in Recently Hospitalized Acutely Depressed Patients. *Neuropsychobiology* 39(2) (Mar 1999):63–70.

94. Barragan-Rodríguez, L., M. Rodríguez-Morán, F. Guerrero-Romero. "Depressive Symptoms and Hypomagnesemia in Older Diabetic Subjects." *Arch Med Res* 38(7) (Oct 2007):752–756.

95. Cundy, T., J. Mackay. "Proton Pump Inhibitors and Severe Hypomagnesemia." *Curr Opin Gastroenterol* 27(2) (Mar 2011):180–185.

96. Nechifor, M. "Magnesium in Major Depression." *Magnes Res* 22(3) (Sep 2009):163S-166S.

97. Jacka, F. N., S. Overland, R. Stewart, et al. "Association Between Magnesium Intake and Depression and Anxiety in Community-Dwelling Adults: The Hordaland Health Study." *Aust N Z J Psychiatry* 43(1) (Jan 2009):45–52.

98. Weston, P. G. "Magnesium as a Sedative." *Am J Psychiatry* 78(4) (Apr 1, 1922): 637–638.

99. Eby, G. A., K. L. Eby. "Rapid Recovery from Major Depression Using Magnesium Treatment." *Med Hypotheses* 67(2) (2006):362–370.

100. Barragán-Rodríguez, L., M. Rodríguez-Morán, F. Guerrero-Romero. "Efficacy and Safety of Oral Magnesium Supplementation in the Treatment of Depression in the Elderly with Type 2 Diabetes: A Randomized, Equivalent Trial." *Magnes Res* 21(4) (Dec 2008):218–223.

101. Eby, G. A. 3rd, K. L. Eby. "Magnesium for Treatment-Resistant Depression: A Review and Hypothesis." *Med Hypotheses* 74(4) (Apr 2010):649–660.

102. Frederickson, C. J., J. Y. Koh, A. I. Bush. "The Neurobiology of Zinc in Health and Disease." *Nat Rev Neurosci* 6(6) (Jun 2005):449–462.

103. Bitanihirwe, B. K. Y., M. G. Cunningham. "Zinc: The Brain's Dark Horse." *Synapse* 63(11) (Nov 2009):1029–1049. Sensi, S. L., P. Paoletti, J. Y. Koh. "The Neurophysiology and Pathology of Brain Zinc." *J Neurosci* 31(45) (Nov 9, 2011): 16076–16085.

104. Levenson, C. W. "Zinc: The New Antidepressant?" *Nutr Rev* 64(1) (Jan 2006):39–42.

105. Little, K. Y., X. Castellanos, L. L. Humphries, et al. "Altered Zinc Metabolism in Mood Disorder Patients." *Biol Psychiatry* 26(6) (Oct 1989):646–648.Maes, M., P. C. D'Haese, S. Scharpé, et al. "Hypozincemia in Depression." *J Affect Disord* 31(2) (Jun 1994):135–140.

106. Maes, M., E. Vandoolaeghe, H. Neels, et al. "Lower Serum Zinc in Major Depression Is a Sensitive Marker of Treatment Resistance and of the Immune/Inflammatory Response in That Illness." *Biol Psychiatry* 42(5) (Sep 1, 1997):349–358. Siwek, M., D. Dudek, M. Schlegel-Zawadzka, et al. "Serum Zinc Level in Depressed Patients During Zinc Supplementation of Imipramine Treatment." *J Affect Disord* 126(3) (Nov 2010):447–452.

107. Wójcik, J., D. Dudek, M. Schlegel-Zawadzka, et al. "Antepartum/Postpartum Depressive Symptoms and Serum Zinc and Magnesium Levels." *Pharmacol Rep* 58(4) (Jul-Aug 2006):571–576.

108. Amani, R., S. Saeidi, Z. Nazari, et al. "Correlation between Dietary Zinc Intakes and Its Serum Levels with Depression Scales in Young Female Students." *Biol Trace Elem Res* 137(2) (Nov 2010):150–158.

109. Maserejian, N. N., S. A. Hall, J. B. McKinlay. "Low Dietary or Supplemental Zinc Is Associated with Depression Symptoms among Women, but Not Men, in a Population-Based Epidemiological Survey." *J Affect Disord* 136(3) (Feb 2012):781–788.

110. Yary, T., S. Aazami. "Dietary Intake of Zinc Was Inversely Associated with Depression." *Biol Trace Elem Res* 145(3) (Mar 2012):286–290.

111. Szewczyk, B., M. Kubera, G. Nowak. "The Role of Zinc in Neurodegenerative Inflammatory Pathways in Depression." *Prog Neuropsychopharmacol Biol Psychiatry* 35(3) (Apr 29, 2011):693–701.

112. Nechifor, M. "Magnesium in Major Depression." *Magnes Res* 22(3) (Sep 2009):163S–166S.

113. Sawada, T., K. Yokoi. "Effect of Zinc Supplementation on Mood States in Young Women: A Pilot Study." *Eur J Clin Nutr* 64(3) (Mar 2010):331–333.

114. Bryce-Smith, D., R. I. Simpson. "Case of Anorexia Nervosa Responding to Zinc Sulphate." *Lancet* 324(8398) (Aug 1984):350.

115. Katz, R. L., C. L. Keen, I. F. Litt, et al. "Zinc Deficiency in Anorexia Nervosa." *J Adolesc Health Care* 8(5) (Sep 1987):400–406.

116. Nowak, G., M. Siwek, D. Dudek, et al. "Effect of Zinc Supplementation on Antidepressant Therapy in Unipolar Depression: A Preliminary Placebo-Controlled Study." *Pol J Pharmacol* 55(6) (Nov-Dec 2003):1143–1147.

117. Siwek, M., D. Dudek, I. A. Paul, et al. "Zinc Supplementation Augments Efficacy of Imipramine in Treatment Resistant Patients: A Double Blind, Placebo-Controlled Study." *J Affect Disord* 118(1–3) (Nov 2009):187–195.

118. Lai, J., A. Moxey, G. Nowak, et al. "The Efficacy of Zinc Supplementation in Depression: Systematic Review of Randomized Controlled Trials." *J Affect Disord* 136(1–2) (Jan 2012):e31–39.

119. Xia, Y., K. E. Hill, P. Li, et al. "Optimization of Selenoprotein P and Other Plasma Selenium Biomarkers for the Assessment of the Selenium Nutritional Requirement:

A Placebo-Controlled, Double-Blind Study of Selenomethionine Supplementation in Selenium-Deficient Chinese Subjects." *Am J Clin Nutr* 92(3) (Jun 23, 2010):525–531.

120. Schrauzer, G. N., P. F. Surai. "Selenium in Human and Animal Nutrition: Resolved and Unresolved Issues. A Partly Historical Treatise in Commemoration of the Fiftieth Anniversary of the Discovery of the Biological Essentiality of Selenium, Dedicated to the Memory of Klaus Scharz (1914–1978) on the Occasion of the Thirtieth Anniversary of His Death." *Crit Rev Biotechnol* 29(1) (2009):2–9.

121. Benton, D. "Selenium Intake, Mood and Other Aspects of Psychological Functioning." *Nutr Neurosci* 5(6) (Dec 2002):363–374.

122. Rayman, M., A. Thompson, M. Warren-Perry, et al. "Impact of Selenium on Mood and Quality of Life: A Randomized, Controlled Trial." *Biol Psychiatry* 59(2) (Jan 15, 2006):147–154.

123. Mokhber, N., M. Namjoo, F. Tara, et al. "Effect of Supplementation with Selenium on Postpartum Depression: A Randomized Double-Blind Placebo-Controlled Trial." *J Matern Fetal Neonatal Med* 24(1) (Jan 2011):104–108.

124. Sher, L. "The Link Between Alcohol Abuse and Suicide: Possible Role of Selenium Deficiency." *Med Hypotheses* 70(4) (2008):899.

125. Krikorian, R., J. C. Eliassen, E. L. Boespflug, et al. "Improved Cognitive-Cerebral Function in Older Adults with Chromium Supplementation." *Nutr Neurosci* 13(3) (Jun 2010):116–122.

126. McLeod, M. N. *Lifting Your Depression: How a Psychiatrist Discovered Chromium's Role in the Treatment of Depression.* 2nd ed. Laguna Beach, CA: Basic Health, 2009.

127. McLeod, M. N. "Chromium Treatment of Depression." *Int J Neuropsychopharmacol* 3(4) (Dec 2000):311–314.

128. Posternak, M. A., M. Zimmerman. "The Prevalence of Atypical Features Across Mood, Anxiety, and Personality Disorders." *Compr Psychiatry* 43(4) (Jul-Aug 2002):253–262.

129. Davidson, J. R., K. Abraham, K. M. Connor, et al. "Effectiveness of Chromium in Atypical Depression: A Placebo-Controlled Trial." *Biol Psychiatry* 53(3) (Feb 1, 2003):261–264.

130. Docherty, J. P., D. A. Sack, M. Roffman, et al. "A Double-Blind, Placebo-Controlled, Exploratory Trial of Chromium Picolinate in Atypical Depression: Effect on Carbohydrate Craving." *J Psychiatr Pract* 11(5) (Sep 2005):302–314.

131. Mouritsen, O. G. *Life—As a Matter of Fat: The Emerging Science of Lipidomics.* Berlin: Springer, 2005. Taubes, G. *Good Calories, Bad Calories: Challenging the Controversial Wisdom on Diet, Weight Control, and Disease.* New York: Knopf, 2007. Ravnskov, U. *Ignore the Awkward! How the Cholesterol Myths are Kept Alive.* CreateSpace, 2010.

132. Asellus, P., P. Nordström, J. Jokinen. "Cholesterol and CSF 5-HIAA in Attempted Suicide." *J Affect Disord* 125(1–3) (Sep 2010):388–392.

133. Wells, A. S., N. W. Read, J. D. Laugharne, et al. "Alterations in Mood after Changing to a Low-Fat Diet." *Br J Nutr* 79(1) (Jan 1998):23–30.

134. Burr, G. O., M. N. Burr. "A New Deficiency Disease Produced by the Rigid Exclusion of Fat from the Diet." *J Biol Chem* 82(2) (1929):345–367.

135. Burr, G. O., M. M. Burr. "On the Nature and Role of the Fatty Acids Essential in Nutrition." *J Biol Chem* 86(2) (1930):587–621.

136. Childs, C. E., M. Romeu-Nadal, G. C. Burdge, et al. "Gender Differences in the *n*-3 Fatty Acid Content of Tissues." *Proc Nutr Soc* 67(1) (Feb 2008):19–27.

137. Brenner, R. R. "Hormonal Modulation of Delta6 and Delta5 Desaturases: Case of Diabetes." *Prostaglandins Leukot Essent Fatty Acids* 68(2) (Feb 2003):151–162.

138. Sinclair, H. M. "Deficiency of Essential Fatty Acids and Atherosclerosis, Etcetera." *Lancet* 270(6919) (Apr 7, 1956):381–383.

139. Ewin, J. *Fine Wines and Fish Oil: The Life of Hugh Macdonald Sinclair.* Oxford: Oxford University Press, 2001.

140. Crawford, M. A., S. Crawford. *What We Eat Today.* London: Spearman, 1972.

141. Horrobin, D. F. "The Roles of Prostaglandins and Prolactin in Depression, Mania and Schizophrenia." *Postgrad Med J* 53(Suppl 4) (1977):160–165.

142. Hibbeln, J. R. "Fish Consumption and Major Depression." *Lancet* 351(9110) (Apr 18, 1998):1213.

143. Hibbeln, J. R. "Seafood Consumption, the DHA Content of Mothers' Milk and Prevalence Rates of Postpartum Depression: A Cross-National, Ecological Analysis." *J Affect Disord* 69(1–3) (May 2002):15–29.

144. Puri, B. K., S. J. Counsell, G. Hamilton, et al. "Eicosapentaenoic Acid in Treatment-Resistant Depression Associated with Symptom Remission, Structural Brain Changes and Reduced Neuronal Phospholipid Turnover." *Int J Clin Pract* 55(8) (Oct 2001):560–563.

145. Chiu, C. C., S. Y. Huang, W. W. Shen, et al. "Omega-3 Fatty Acids for Depression in Pregnancy." *Am J Psychiatry* 160(2) (2003):385.

146. Sublette, M. E., S. P. Ellis, A. L. Geant, et al. "Meta-Analysis of the Effects of Eicosapentaenoic Acid (EPA) in Clinical Trials in Depression." *J Clin Psychiatry* 72(12) (Dec 2011):1577–1584.

147. Simopoulos, A. P. "Omega-3 Fatty Acids in Inflammation and Autoimmune Diseases." *J Am Coll Nutr* 21(6) (Dec 2002):495–505.

148. Dowlati, Y., N. Herrmann, W. Swardfager, et al. "A Meta-analysis of Cytokines in Major Depression." *Biol Psychiatry* 67(5) (Mar 1, 2010):446–457.

149. Pascoe, M. C., S. G. Crewther, L. M. Carey, et al. "What You Eat Is What You Are—A Role for Polyunsaturated Fatty acids in Neuroinflammation Induced Depression?" *Clin Nutr* 30(4) (Aug 2011):407–415.

150. Perica, M. M., Delas, I. "Essential Fatty Acids and Psychiatric Disorders." *Nutr Clin Pract* 26(4) (Aug 2011):409–425.

151. Saravanan, P., N. C. Davidson, E. B. Schmidt, et al. "Cardiovascular Effects of Marine Omega-3 Fatty Acids." *Lancet* 376(9740) (Aug 14, 2010):540–550.

152. Calder, P. C. "Fatty Acids and Inflammation: The Cutting Edge Between Food and Pharma." *Eur J Pharmacol* 668(Suppl 1) (Sep 2011):S50-S58.

153. Altschuler, L. L., M. Bauer, M. A. Frye, et al. "Does Thyroid Supplementation Accelerate Tricyclic Antidepressant Response? A Review and Meta-Analysis of the Literature." *Am J Psychiatry* 158(10) (Oct 2001):1617–1622.

154. Bauer, M., R. Hellweg, K. J. Gräf, et al. "Treatment of Refractory Depression with High-Dose Thyroxine." *Neuropsychopharmacology* 18(6) (Jun 1998):444–455.

Chapter 9: Multinutrient Treatment

1. Gerson, M. *A Cancer Therapy: Results of Fifty Cases.* 3rd ed. Del Mar, CA: Totality Books, 1975.

2. Saul, A. W. "Hidden in Plain Sight: The Pioneering Work of Frederick Robert Klenner, M.D." *J Orthomol Med* 22(1) (2007):31–38.

3. Kaufman, W. *The Common Form of Joint Dysfunction: Its Incidence and Treatment.* Brattleboro, VT: Hildreth & Co, 1949.

4. Schuitemaker, G. E., A. J. Hoogland. "Cobalamin Deficiency, Methylation and Neurological Disorders." *J Orthomol Med* 11(4th Quarter) (1996):190–194. Mitchell, J. A. "The Effect of Folic Acid and B_{12} on Depression: Twelve Case Studies." *J Orthomol Med* 22(4) (2007):183–192.

5. Cheng, T., Z. Zhu, S. Masuda, et al. "Effects of Multinutrient Supplementation on Antioxidant Defense Systems in Healthy Human Beings." *J Nutr Biochem* 12(7) (Jul 2001):388–395.

6. Ames, B. N. "Supplements and Tuning Up Metabolism." *J Nutr* 134(11) (2004):3164S–3168S.

7. Ames, B. N. "Low Micronutrient Intake May Accelerate the Degenerative Diseases of Aging through Allocation of Scarce Micronutrients by Triage." *Proc Natl Acad Sci USA* 103(47) (Nov 21, 2006):17589–17594.

8. Benton, D., J. Haller, J. Fordy. "Vitamin Supplementation for 1 Year Improves Mood." *Neuropsychobiology* 32(2) (1995):98–105.

9. Bell, I. R., J. S. Edman, F. D. Morrow, et al. "Brief Communication. Vitamin B_1, B_2, and B_6 Augmentation of Tricyclic Antidepressant Treatment in Geriatric Depression with Cognitive Dysfunction." *J Am Coll Nutr* 11(2) (Apr 1992):159–163.

10. Kennedy, D. O., R. Veasey, A. Watson, et al. "Effects of High-Dose B Vitamin Complex with Vitamin C and Minerals on Subjective Mood and Performance in Healthy Males." *Psychopharmacology (Berl)* 211(1) (Jul 2010):55–68.

11. Harris, E., J. Kirk, R. Rowsell, et al. "The Effect of Multivitamin Supplementation on Mood and Stress in Healthy Older Men." *Hum Psychopharmacol* 26(8) (Dec 2011):560–567.

12. Maes, M., Z. Fisar, M. Medina, et al. "New Drug Targets in Depression: Inflammatory, Cell-Mediated Immune, Oxidative and Nitrosative Stress, Mitochondrial, Antioxidant, and Neuroprogressive Pathways. And New Drug Candidates—Nrf2 Activators and GSK-3 Inhibitors." *Inflammopharmacology* 20(3) (Jun 2012):127–150.

13. Dunn-Lewis, C., W. J. Kraemer, B. R. Kupchak, et al. "A Multi-Nutrient Supplement Reduced Markers of Inflammation and Improved Physical Performance in Active

Individuals of Middle to Older Age: A Randomized, Double-Blind, Placebo-Controlled Study." *Nutr J* 10 (Sep 7, 2011):90.

14. Schmitz, S. M., J. E. Hofheins, R. Lemieux. "Nine Weeks of Supplementation with a Multi-Nutrient Product Augments Gains in Lean Mass, Strength, and Muscular Performance in Resistance Trained Men." *J Int Soc Sports Nutr* 7 (Dec 16, 2010):40.

15. Stratton, R. J., M. Elia. "Encouraging Appropriate, Evidence-Based Use of Oral Nutritional Supplements." *Proc Nutr Soc* 69(4) (Nov 2010):477–487.

16. Kamphuis, P. J., P. Scheltens. "Can Nutrients Prevent or Delay Onset of Alzheimer's Disease?" *J Alzheimers Dis* 20(3) (2010):765–775.

17. Öckerman, P. A. "Improvement of Arterial Stiffness by Multi-Nutrient Supplementation." *J Orthomol Med* 26(4) (2011):159–162.

18. Gaby, A. "Nutritional Treatments for Acute Myocardial Infarction." *Altern Med Rev* 15(2) (Jul 2010):113–123.

19. Houston, M. C. "The Role of Cellular Micronutrient Analysis, Nutraceuticals, Vitamins, Antioxidants and Minerals in the Prevention and Treatment of Hypertension and Cardiovascular Disease." *Ther Adv Cardiovasc Dis* 4(3) (Jun 2010):165–183.

20. Davidson, J. R., C. Crawford, J. A. Ives, et al. "Homeopathic Treatments in Psychiatry: A Systematic Review of Randomized Placebo-Controlled Studies." *J Clin Psychiatry* 72(6) (Jun 2011):795–805.

21. Adler, U. C., N. M. P. Paiva, A. T. Cesar, et al. "Homeopathic Individualized Q-Potencies versus Fluoxetine for Moderate to Severe Depression: Double-Blind, Randomized Non-Inferiority Trial." *Evid Based Complement Alternat Med* 2011:520182. (Jun 8, 2011) Epub.

Chapter 10: Bipolar Disorder

1. de Freitas, D. M., M. M. Castro, C. F. Geraldes. "Is Competition between Li+ and Mg2+ the Underlying Theme in the Proposed Mechanisms for the Pharmacological Action of Lithium Salts in Bipolar Disorder?" *Acc Chem Res* 39(4) (Apr 2006): 283–291. Dudev, T., C. Lim, C. "Competition between Li+ and Mg2+ in metalloproteins. Implications for lithium therapy." *J Am Chem Soc* 133(24) (2011):9506–9515.

2. Gardner, R. Jr. "Mechanisms in Manic-Depressive Disorder: An Evolutionary Model." *Arch Gen Psychiatry* 39(12) (Dec 1982):1436–1441.

3. Wehr, T. A., W. C. Duncan Jr., L. Sher, et al. "A Circadian Signal of Change of Season in Patients with Seasonal Affective Disorder." *Arch Gen Psychiatry* 58(12) (Dec 2001):1108–1114.

4. Kretschmer, E. *Physique and Character. An Investigation of the Nature of Constitution and of the Theory of Temperament.* New York: Harcourt, Brace & Company, 1925.

5. Sherman, J. A. "Evolutionary Origin of Bipolar Disorder–Revised: EOBD-R." *Med Hypotheses* 78(1) (Jan 2012):113–122.

6. Andreasen, N. C., I. D. Glick. "Bipolar Affective Disorder and Creativity: Implications and Clinical Management." *Compr Psychiatry* 29(3) (May-Jun 1988):207–217. Andreasen, N. C. "The Relationship between Creativity and Mood Disorders." *Dia-*

logues Clin Neurosci 10(2) (2008):251–255. Kyaga, S., P. Lichtenstein, M. Boman, et al. "Creativity and Mental Disorder: Family Study of 300,000 People with Severe Mental Disorder." *Br J Psychiatry* 199(5) (Nov 2011):373–379.

7. Stoll, A. L., W. E. Severus, M. P. Freeman, et al. "Omega-3 Fatty Acids in Bipolar Disorder: A Preliminary Double-Blind, Placebo-Controlled Trial." *Arch Gen Psychiatry* 56(5) (May 1999):407–412.

8. Sarris, J., D. Mischoulon, I. Schweitzer. "Omega-3 for Bipolar Disorder: Meta-Analyses of Use in Mania and Bipolar Depression." *J Clin Psychiatry* 73(1) (Jan 2012):81–86.

9. Coppen, A., S. Chaudhry, C. Swade. "Folic Acid Enhances Lithium Profylaxis." *J Affect Disord* 10(1) (Jan-Feb 1986):9–13.

10. Berk, M., D. L. Copolov, O. Dean, et al. "N-Acetyl Cysteine for Depressive Symptoms in Bipolar Disorder—A Double-Blind Randomized Placebo-Controlled Trial." *Biol Psychiatry* 64(6) (Sep 15, 2008):468–475. Berk, M., O. Dean, S. M. Cotton, et al. "The Efficacy of N-Acetylcysteine as an Adjunctive Treatment in Bipolar Depression: An Open Label Trial." *J Affect Disord* 135(1–3) (Dec 2011):389–394.

11. Giannini, A. J., A. M. Nakoneczie, S. M. Melemis, et al. "Magnesium Oxide Augmentation of Verapamil Maintenance Therapy in Mania." *Psychiatry Res* 93(1) (Feb 14, 2000):83–87.

12. Szewczyk, B., A. Palucha-Poniewiera, E. Poleszak, et al. "Investigational NMDA Receptor Modulators for Depression." *Expert Opin Investig Drugs* 21(1) (Jan 2012):91–102.

13. Pasquali, L., C. L. Busceti, F. Fulceri, et al. "Intracellular Pathways Underlying the Effects of Lithium." *Behav Pharmacol* 21(5–6) (Sep 2010):473–492.

14. Behzadi, A. H., Z. Omrani, M. Chalian, et al. "Folic Acid Efficacy as an Alternative Drug Added to Sodium Valproate in the Treatment of Acute Phase of Mania in Bipolar Disorder: A Double-Blind Randomized Controlled Trial." *Acta Psychiatr Scand* 120(6) (Dec 2009):441–445.

15. Sarris, J., D. Mischoulon, I. Schweitzer. "Adjunctive Nutraceuticals with Standard Pharmacotherapies in Bipolar Disorder: A Systematic Review of Clinical Trials." *Bipolar Disord* 13(5–6) (Aug–Sep 2011):454–465. Sarris, J., J. Lake, R. Hoenders. "Bipolar Disorder and Complementary Medicine: Current Evidence, Safety Issues, and Clinical Considerations." *J Altern Complement Med* 17(10) (Oct 2011):881–890.

16. Berk, M., P. Conus, F. Kapczinski, et al. "From Neuroprogression to Neuroprotection: Implications for Clinical Care." *Med J Aust* 193(4 Suppl) (Aug 16, 2010):S36–S40. Berk, M., F. Kapczinski, A. C. Andreazza, et al. "Pathways Underlying Neuroprogression in Bipolar Disorder: Focus on Inflammation, Oxidative Stress and Neurotrophic Factors." *Neurosci Biobehav Rev* 35(3) (Jan 2011):804–817.

17. Kato, T., N. Kato. "Mitochondrial Dysfunction in Bipolar Disorder." *Bipolar Disord* 2(3 Pt 1) (Sep 2000):180–190. Stork, C., P. F. Renshaw. "Mitochondrial Dysfunction in Bipolar Disorder: Evidence from Magnetic Resonance Spectroscopy Research." *Mol Psychiatry* 10(10) (Oct 2005):900–919.

18. Aw, T. Y., D. P. Jones. "Nutrients Supply and Mitochondrial Function." *Annu Rev Nutr* 9 (1989):229–251. Cohen, B. H., D. R. Gold. "Mitochondrial Cytopathy in Adults: What We Know So Far." *Cleve Clin J Med* 68(7) (Jul 2001):625–642. Ames,

B. N., H. Atamna, D. W. Killilea. "Mineral and Vitamin Deficiencies Can Accelerate the Mitochondrial Decay of Aging." *Mol Aspects Med* 26(4–5) (Jul 2005):363–378. Pieczenik, S. R., J. Neustadt. "Mitochondrial Dysfunction and Molecular Pathways of Disease." *Exp Mol Pathol* 83(1) (Aug 2007):84–92.

19. Hoffer, A. "Bipolar Disorder and Orthomolecular Treatment." *Townsend Letter* 317 (2009):44–50.

20. Truehope Nutritional Support, Ltd. website, http://www.truehope.com.

21. Kaplan, B. J., J. S. Simpson, R. C. Ferre, et al. "Effective Mood Stabilization in Bipolar Disorder with a Chelated Mineral Supplement." *J Clin Psychiatry* 62(12) (Dec 2001):936–944.

22. Frazier, E. A., M. A. Fristad, L. E. Arnold. "Multinutrient Supplement as Treatment: Literature Review and Case Report of a 12-Year-Old Boy with Bipolar Disorder." *J Child Adolesc Psychopharmacol* 19(4) (Aug 2009):453–460.

23. Gately, D., B. J. Kaplan. "Database Analysis of Adults with Bipolar Disorder Consuming a Micronutrient Formula." *Clin Med: Psychiatry* 4 (2009):3–16.

24. Jacka, F. N., J. A. Pasco, A. Mykletun, et al. "Diet Quality in Bipolar Disorder in a Population-Based Sample of Women." *J Affect Disord* 129(1–3) (Mar 2011):332–337.

25. Frank, E. *Treating Bipolar Disorder: A Clinician's Guide to Interpersonal and Social Rhythm Therapy.* New York: Guilford Press, 2007.

Chapter 12. Unstress and Un-Depress Your Life

1. Chiesa, A., Serretti, A. "Mindfulness Based Cognitive Therapy for Psychiatric Disorders: A Systematic Review and Meta-Analysis." *Psychiatry Res* 187:3 (2011): 441–453.

Chapter 13. Depression: Observations and Comments

1. Taylor, Jill Bolte. *My Stroke of Insight: A Brain Scientist's Personal Journey.* New York: Viking, 2008.

INDEX

ABOUT THE AUTHORS

Bo H. Jonsson, M.D., Ph.D., has been a practicing psychiatrist for thirty years. He studied medicine at Lund University and later at the Karolinska Institutet in Stockholm, where he received his medical degree and wrote his medical dissertation. He is affiliated with the Department of Clinical Neuroscience, Section of Psychiatry, Karolinska Institutet. Currently he is medical director of Center for Affective disorders, Northern Stockholm Psychiatry, St Göran's Hospital, Stockholm. Dr. Jonsson is on the editorial board of the *Journal of Orthomolecular Medicine,* and is president of the Swedish Society for Orthomolecular Medicine.

Andrew W. Saul, M.S., Ph.D., is Editor-in-chief of the Orthomolecular Medicine News Service and is on the editorial board of the Journal of Orthomolecular Medicine. He has published over 175 peer-reviewed articles and has written a dozen books. He was on the faculty of the State University of New York for nine years, and has twice won New York Empire State Fellowships for teaching. *Psychology Today* magazine named him one of seven natural health pioneers, and he is featured in the documentary movie *Food Matters.* His website, Doctor Yourself.com, is the largest non-commercial natural healing resource on the Internet.

www.ingramcontent.com/pod-product-compliance
Lightning Source LLC
Jackson TN
JSHW011358130125
77033JS00023B/742

* 9 7 8 1 5 9 1 2 0 2 8 2 0 *